CLINICAL GI PHYSIOLOGY FOR THE EXAM TAKER

Eugene D. Jacobson, M.D.
Professor of Medicine and Physiology
The University of Colorado Health Sciences Center School of Medicine
Denver, Colorado

Joel S. Levine, M.D.
Professor of Medicine
The University of Colorado Health Sciences Center School of Medicine
Denver, Colorado

W.B. SAUNDERS COMPANY
A Division of Harcourt Brace & Company
PHILADELPHIA   LONDON   TORONTO   MONTREAL   SYDNEY   TOKYO

W.B. SAUNDERS COMPANY
A Division of
Harcourt Brace & Company

The Curtis Center
Independence Square West
Philadelphia, Pennsylvania 19106

Library of Congress Cataloging-in-Publication Data

Jacobson, Eugene D.
  Clinical GI physiology for the exam taker / Eugene D. Jacobson, Joel S. Levine.
    p.   cm.
  ISBN 0-7216-3701-9
  1. Gastrointestinal system – Physiology. 2. Gastrointestinal system – Pathophysiology. I. Levine, Joel S.
(Joel Seth). II. Title. III. Title: Clinical gastrointestinal physiology for the exam taker.
  [DNLM: 1. Gastrointestinal System – physiology – examination questions. WI 18 J17c 1994]
  QP145.J36 1994
  612.3'2'076 – dc20
  DNLM/DLC   93 - 8348

CLINICAL GI PHYSIOLOGY FOR THE EXAM TAKER   ISBN 0-7216-3701-9

Copyright © 1994 by W.B. Saunders Company

All rights reserved. No part of this publication may be reproduced or transmitted in any form or by any means, electronic or mechanical, including photocopy, recording, or any information storage and retrieval system, without permission in writing from the publisher.

Printed in the United States of America

Last digit is the print number: 9   8   7   6   5   4   3   2   1

PREFACE

We are committed teachers who love our work. An important segment of the people whom we are privileged to teach are advanced medical professionals such as gastroenterology fellows, general surgery residents, and young practicing gastroenterologists in the community. Their devotion to learning, their energy and enthusiasm, and their prospects for the future have been an inspiration to us. This book is dedicated to them.

These three groups of advanced professionals also share the challenge and the burden of imminent comprehensive examinations that will have a bearing on their future prospects and careers. Gastroenterology fellows are usually less than 2 years away from board examinations in their specialty; general surgery residents have inservice examinations annually; and community gastroenterologists certified since 1990 have recertification examinations every 5 years. Second-year medical students preparing for National Board examinations may find this text useful.

Although the major topical component of such examinations is clinical gastroenterology or general surgery, a significant lesser component is the basic science that underlies the clinical field, especially gastrointestinal physiology and pathophysiology. This book addresses these critical areas for the advanced professional who will shortly be wrestling with examination questions about gastrointestinal functions and dysfunctions. In this book, gastrointestinal physiology and pathophysiology have been organized into eight chapters dealing with motility; gastric secretion; pancreatic secretion; intestinal salt and water transport; digestion and absorption of carbohydrates and proteins, lipids, and minerals and vitamins; and splanchnic circulation.

Each chapter considers physiology as it relates to underlying mechanisms and overall control of specific functions. There is also a balance between cell biology, which is usually the realm of mechanisms, and integrative biology, which is usually the setting for control of organ functions.

The format of each chapter is unique for a text focusing on the basic science of gastroenterology. Each chapter begins with a case report of a patient whose illness exemplifies derangements in the physiology constituting the major topic of the chapter. This is followed by the body of the chapter, in which the physiology and pathophysiology are described. Then, the original case report is resumed for consideration of diagnosis and management. The chapter concludes with an overview of the illness and an explanation of how the clinical story expresses main points in the physiological topic.

Each chapter is succinct yet solidly based on current levels of widely held scientific and clinical knowledge. This is a readable text and not an outline. Its length is such that a chapter can be read meaningfully in less than 2 hours by an advanced professional. Some of the information in this brief book will refresh the memory of its intended audience, and some information will be new.

The illustrations are also unique for a book of this type. We believe the reader will find them helpful in conceptualizing major points in the text. We are indebted to our publisher, Lewis Reines, who convinced us to use color diagrams to visualize and emphasize information, and we are especially grateful to Mollie Dunker, whose skills and artistry have created nearly 90 such visual highlights. We also wish to express our appreciation to Dr. Geza Remak, who carefully scrutinized many of the chapters in this book during their formative stages and shared his criticisms to improve the text. Finally, we are indebted to Kathleen Fernandez, who spent many, many hours carefully retyping the numerous iterations of the text in this book.

CONTENTS

CHAPTER ONE • *Gastrointestinal Motility* 1

CHAPTER TWO • *Gastric Secretion* **25**

CHAPTER THREE • *Pancreatic Secretion* **45**

CHAPTER FOUR • *Intestinal Transport of Salt and Water* **57**

CHAPTER FIVE • *Digestion and Absorption of Carbohydrates and Proteins* **73**

CHAPTER SIX • *Digestion and Absorption of Lipids* **83**

CHAPTER SEVEN • *Mineral and Vitamin Absorption* **93**

CHAPTER EIGHT • *Splanchnic Circulation* **105**

INDEX • **127**

CHAPTER ONE

Gastrointestinal Motility

CASE REPORTS: INITIAL INFORMATION

• Case 1 •

A 37-year-old woman was referred to you for evaluation because of episodic chest pain during the past 2 years. She was married, had three children, drank eight cups of coffee and one or two beers each day, and smoked 1½ packs of cigarettes daily. She was well until 2 years ago, when she developed a substernal, pressure-like pain while watching television. The pain radiated into her neck, was associated with diaphoresis, lasted about 30 min, and then remitted spontaneously. Over the next year, the patient had eight similar episodes and finally went to an emergency room when she was awakened from sleep by the pain. There was no clear association with eating, exercise, or body position. She felt completely well between attacks, with no heartburn, dysphagia, shortness of breath, odynophagia, cough, pleurisy, hemoptysis, or palpitations. Her family history was negative for cardiac and gastrointestinal diseases, and she was not using prescribed medications or cocaine. Her pain had stopped by the time she reached the emergency department.

The patient was 5 feet 4 inches tall and weighed 185 lb. Her physical examination in the emergency department was normal except for obesity and scattered rhonchi in the lungs that cleared with a cough. There was no chest wall tenderness, abnormal heart sounds (clicks, murmurs), or blood in the stool. The electrocardiogram was normal. The patient was encouraged to stop drinking coffee and smoking cigarettes, referred to a cardiologist, and given sublingual nitroglycerin (NTG) to take if the pain recurred. The patient followed none of these recommendations until her third subsequent attack 5 months later.

At this time her history and physical examination were unchanged, and the cardiologist sequentially obtained an exercise cardiogram, an exercise thallium scan, and an echocardiogram, all of which were normal. Because of continued episodes of pain, which were prolonged to 45 to 60 min despite NTG, the patient underwent a cardiac catheterization; the coronary arteries were normal and did not go into spasm after administration of edrophonium.

Referral to a gastroenterologist led to an esophagogram, an upper gastrointestinal endoscopy with biopsies of the esophagus, and an esophageal motility test. Only the last test was abnormal. About 20 percent of the contraction waves in the esophagus were simultaneous rather than peristaltic, of high pressure (110 mm Hg), and of long (4 sec) duration. Edrophonium increased the proportion of abnormal contractions. The patient did not experience pain during the study. Subsequently the patient was placed on a long-acting nitrate and a calcium channel antagonist but stopped each after 2 weeks because of side effects (i.e., headache with the nitrate and constipation with the calcium channel antagonist). Because of the recurrence of pain, she was referred for your opinion as to the advisability of an esophageal myotomy for her problem.

• Case 2 •

A 26-year-old woman sought your evaluation of her lifelong constipation. Since childhood she could not remember experiencing a spontaneous bowel movement. About every 2 to 3 days her mother gave her an enema and about once a month, castor oil. As a teenager she extended the time between enemas to every 7 to 10 days. She never felt the urge to defecate, and abdominal bloating invariably led to the use of an enema. Her feces were hard and pebble-like. Her diet contained essentially no fiber, as any cereals or fresh fruits or vegetables (or psyllium) worsened the bloating sensation. She denied laxative use, binge eating, induced vomiting, weight loss, excessive exercise, sexual or physical abuse as a child, or any health problems other than the constipation.

The patient, an executive secretary, was married with no children, and did not smoke or drink alcoholic beverages. Her mother and maternal grandmother had had constipation for most of their lives and took enemas or laxatives. There was no other pertinent family history.

The physical examination revealed normal vital signs, a weight of 104 lb, a height of 5 feet 6 inches, a slightly distended abdomen, and a slightly tender left lower quadrant without masses or organomegaly. A rectal examination revealed hard stool in the rectal vault; a Hemoccult test was negative. The neurological examination was normal.

PHYSIOLOGY

Gastrointestinal motility refers to the mechanical movements of the muscular walls of the hollow digestive organs. These motor activities serve several important functions in the gastrointestinal tract. First, propulsive motor activity moves food and digestive juices from the mouth to the small bowel, where most nutrient digestion takes place. Propulsion is also required to move undigestible materials into the colon and fecal material through the anus to the outside. Second, motility is essential to mix ingested nutrients with digestive juices. This churning facilitates the chemical and physical dissolution of nutrients preparatory to their absorption. Movements of the mucosal lining of the lumen also expose more surface area for the absorption of digested nutrients and water. Finally, because of its ability to relax, the visceral smooth muscle wall accommodates to luminal contents and permits protracted storage of those contents in the proximal stomach and colon. As a result of the foregoing motor activities, the other major functions of the gastrointestinal tract—namely, secretion, digestion, absorption, and excretion—reach optimal levels.

Motility is controlled mostly by involuntary factors—namely, the autonomic nerves and the contractile properties of visceral smooth muscle. Part of the autonomic nervous control is extrinsic to the digestive organs and part is contained in intrinsic networks, primarily in the intramural myenteric and submucosal neural plexuses. The intrinsic nerves are often referred to as the "enteric nervous system."

The extrinsic parasympathetic innervation of the digestive organs is contained primarily in preganglionic efferent fibers of the vagus nerves. The vagi innervate the esophagus, stomach, small intestine, and proximal two-thirds of the colon. The pelvic nerves supply parasympathetic efferent fibers to the distal colon and the rectum. Parasympathetic nerves release acetylcholine, which enhances propulsive motility by increasing the frequency and strength of muscular contractions and by relaxing the various sphincters between organs.

The sympathetic component of the autonomic nerves to the gastrointestinal tract is contained in the postganglionic splanchnic nerves, which follow the celiac, superior mesenteric, and inferior mesenteric arteries to their respective abdominal organs. Sympathetic nerves release mainly norepinephrine, which inhibits gastrointestinal motor activity. Although motor responses to the sympathetic system oppose responses to the parasympathetic system, sympathetic effects do not influence gastrointestinal motility as much as do parasympathetic or enteric nervous system effects. The enteric nervous system is located in the walls of the hollow organs, releases acetylcholine and other neurotransmitter agents such as neuropeptides, and is at least as important in regulating motility as the extrinsic parasympathetic system.

Smooth Muscle Cell Contractility

Motility involves contractions and relaxations of the muscular walls of the tubular organs of the digestive system. The walls of these hollow organs are composed mostly of visceral smooth muscle cells. However, striated muscle lines the oropharynx, the proximal one third of the esophagus, and the distal anal canal. A smooth muscle cell is cigar shaped, with dimensions of about 100×10 μm (Fig. 1–1). Some of its distinguishing features related to contractility include intracellular filaments, which contain contractile proteins (myosin and actin), and subcellular structures (sarcoplasmic reticulum and caveolae), which store and release Ca^{++}.

Contraction of a gastrointestinal smooth muscle cell is initiated by a stimulating agonist such as acetylcholine, which binds to its receptor on the plasmalemma of the cell (Fig. 1–2). This step stimulates a G protein at the membrane. G proteins are a family of proteins located in or near cell membranes that can attract high-energy compounds to activate key cytosolic enzymes. In this case the G protein utilizes guanosine triphosphate (GTP) to energize phospholipase C, which converts phosphatidylinositol biphosphate into inositol triphosphate. Several changes then coincide to increase the cytosolic concentration of Ca^{++}:

1. Release of bound Ca^{++} from the sarcoplasmic reticulum and caveolae, mediated by inositol triphosphate.
2. Increased permeability of Ca^{++} channels in the plasmalemma, which accelerates the slow inward Ca^{++} diffusion from the extracellular space into the cytosol.
3. Reduced activity of membrane-bound Ca^{++}–adenosine triphosphatase (Ca^{++}-ATPase), which extrudes the ion from the cell into the extracellular space and into the intracellular storage sites.
4. Electrical depolarization of the plasmalemma, which also increases Ca^{++} diffusion into the cell.

The end result of these interrelated changes is an increase in the concentration of Ca^{++} in the cytosol.

An intracellular protein, calmodulin, quickly binds the Ca^{++} (Fig. 1–3A). Then, the Ca^{++}-calmodulin complex activates myosin kinase, which facilitates the phosphorylation of myosin. Each molecule of myosin receives two high-energy phosphate bonds from adenosine triphosphate (ATP). Lastly, phosphorylated myosin and actin interact to cause

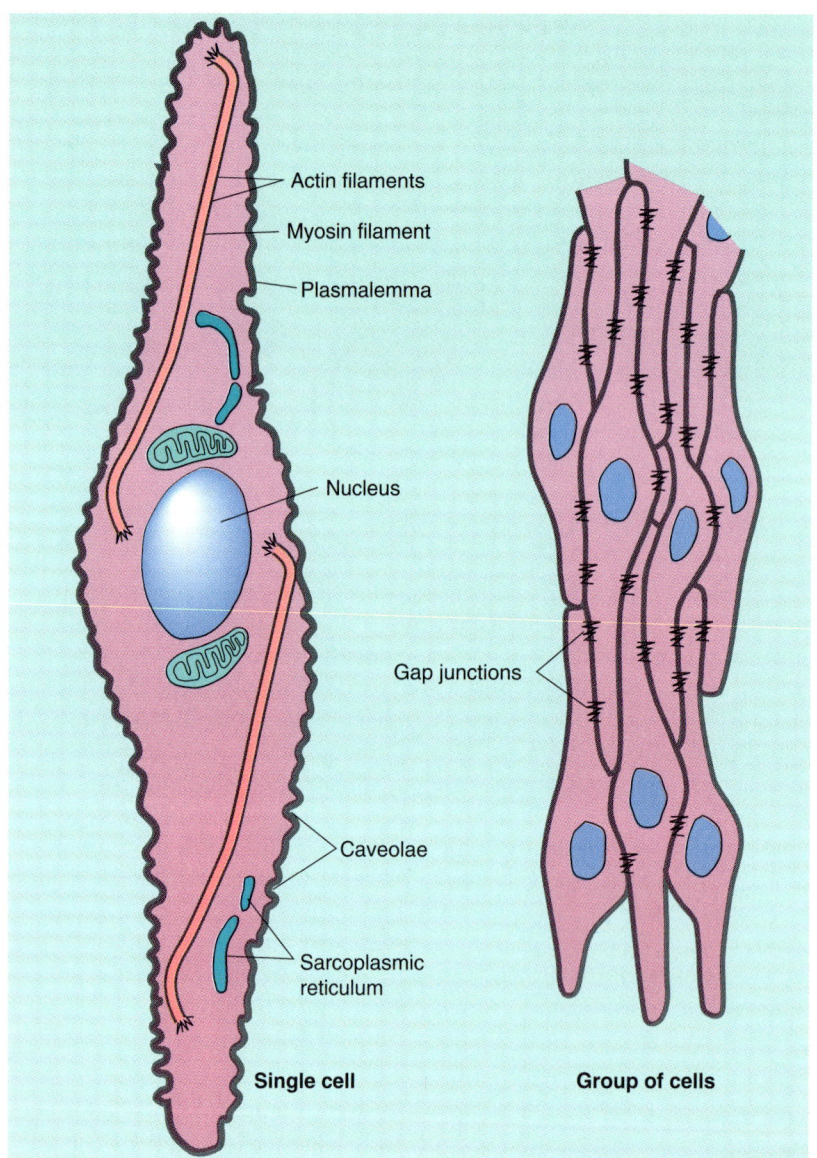

FIGURE 1–1. Visceral smooth muscle cells contain contractile filaments and structures that store calcium. Such cells are connected by gap junctions. The contractile proteins actin and myosin are located in the filaments, and calcium is bound in the sarcoplasmic reticulum and caveolae until the muscle cell contracts. Each smooth muscle cell is connected at its gap junctions to multiple other muscle cells.

cellular contraction. The reverse process—namely, relaxation of the smooth muscle cell—involves restoration of membrane impermeability to extracellular Ca^{++}, activation of Ca^{++}-ATPase to pump the ion out of the cell or into its intracellular storage sites, and hyperpolarization of the plasmalemma. As the cytosolic Ca^{++} concentration decreases, there is less Ca^{++}-calmodulin available, and myosin kinase is deactivated (Fig. 1–3B). Myosin phosphatase then removes the phosphate bonds from myosin, and the muscle cell relaxes.

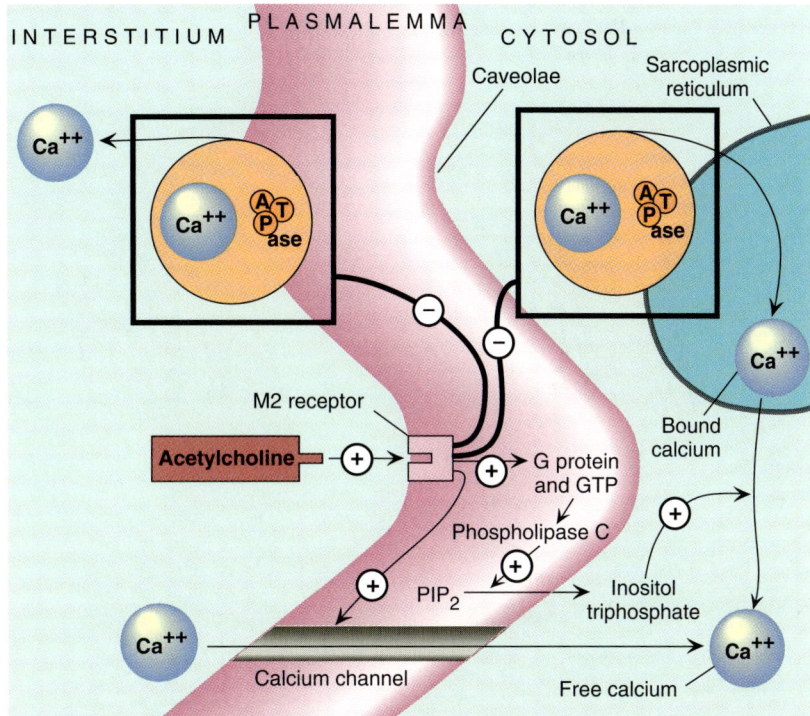

FIGURE 1–2. A smooth muscle stimulant increases intracellular Ca^{++} concentration. A stimulant such as acetylcholine binds to the muscarinic (M_2) receptor on the plasma membrane of the smooth muscle cell and increases the cytosolic [Ca^{++}]. The stimulant opens Ca^{++} channels, thereby accelerating Ca^{++} diffusion from the interstitium. Acetylcholine also stimulates conversion of phosphatidylinositol biphosphate (PIP_2) into inositol triphosphate, an intracellular second messenger that releases bound calcium from intracellular storage sites. Finally, the muscle stimulant inhibits the Ca^{++}–adenosine triphosphatase (Ca^{++}-ATPase) from lowering the cytosolic [Ca^{++}].

Smooth muscle cells are attached to adjacent cells at their respective gap junctions, where fusion of the membranes from different cells occurs (see Fig. 1–1). Many smooth muscle cells are contained in a single muscle bundle surrounded by connective tissue. This organization of smooth muscle cells relative to one another offers two functional advantages. First, a small number of nerves entering a bundle activate a large number of muscle cells because of the coupling of each cell to several nearby cells. The gap junctions are areas of low electrical resistance that permit one excited cell to depolarize multiple neighboring cells. Second, the cells of a bundle contract concurrently, and the bundle behaves as a unit, thereby maximizing the force of its contraction.

Typically, most bundles of smooth muscle cells are further organized in the muscularis of the wall into two functionally separate layers. The inner circular layer's axis is in the circumference of the cavity of the organ, whereas the outer longitudinal layer's axis parallels the length of the hollow organ. In different forms of motor activity, the circular muscle layer can contract either independently of the longitudinal layer (as in segmentation movements of the small bowel) or in a coordinated manner with longitudinal muscle (as in peristalsis).

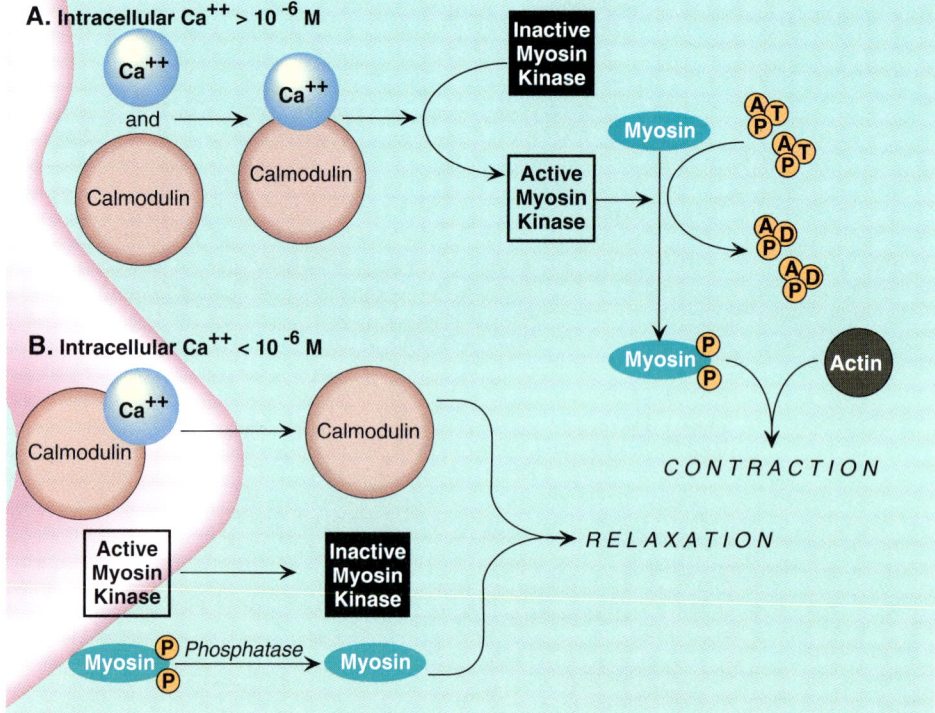

FIGURE 1–3. Intracellular Ca^{++} concentration determines whether visceral smooth muscle contracts or relaxes. When the cytosolic $[Ca^{++}]$ exceeds 10^{-6} mol calmodulin binds Ca^{++} in a complex, thereby activating myosin kinase to facilitate the phosphorylation of myosin by adenosine triphosphate (ATP). Myosin $\sim 2P$ interacts with actin to cause muscle cell contraction. When the intracellular $[Ca^{++}]$ falls below 10^{-6} (as occurs after a contraction or in response to a muscle relaxant, such as vasoactive intestinal peptide), the calmodulin-Ca^{++} complex fails to form, myosin kinase is inactivated, myosin $\sim 2P$ is dephosphorylated, and the cell relaxes.

Mouth and Pharynx

Chewing facilitates ingestion of food but is not essential for digestion. Chewing is normally voluntary but does have an involuntary component. Thus, food placed in the mouth of a brain-injured, comatose patient may initiate a chewing reflex.

Swallowing is the initial major example of motility in the digestive system. The purpose of swallowing is to move food from the mouth into the stomach, and the process involves muscular structures in the oropharynx, esophagus, and upper part of the stomach. Propulsion of solid and liquid food during this set of motor events requires peristaltic movements. Peristalsis is a coordinated sequence of contractions in the wall of a hollow organ. In peristalsis, a band of circular muscle contracts at one point on the wall of the organ, producing an indentation in the wall; then a segment of longitudinal muscle just distal to the indentation contracts, thereby pulling the indentation in the distal direction. Next, the first band of circular muscle relaxes, while the next distal band of circular muscle contracts; after this the first segment of longitudinal muscle relaxes, and then the next distal segment of longitudinal muscle contracts, again pulling the indentation further distally. These contractions can be repeated in a smooth sequence over long stretches of the wall of the hollow organ, giving the appearance of a contractile wave moving slowly in a distal direction. Typical peristaltic waves occur in the oropharynx, esophagus, stomach, small intestine, and rectum.

Swallowing is initiated voluntarily and then becomes completely involuntary. The prime function of the oropharyngeal phase of swallowing is to get the food or liquid into the esophagus without forcing it into the nasopharynx or trachea (Fig. 1–4). The tongue is elevated against the hard palate and then retracts, pushing the food back and forcing the soft palate up against the superior pharyngeal muscle, which contracts, closing the entry to the nasopharynx. The food pushes the epiglottis downward over the trachea, and the glottis is contracted upward to meet the epiglottis, thereby sealing off the trachea from the food. Respiration ceases momentarily. As the bolus of food comes in contact with the

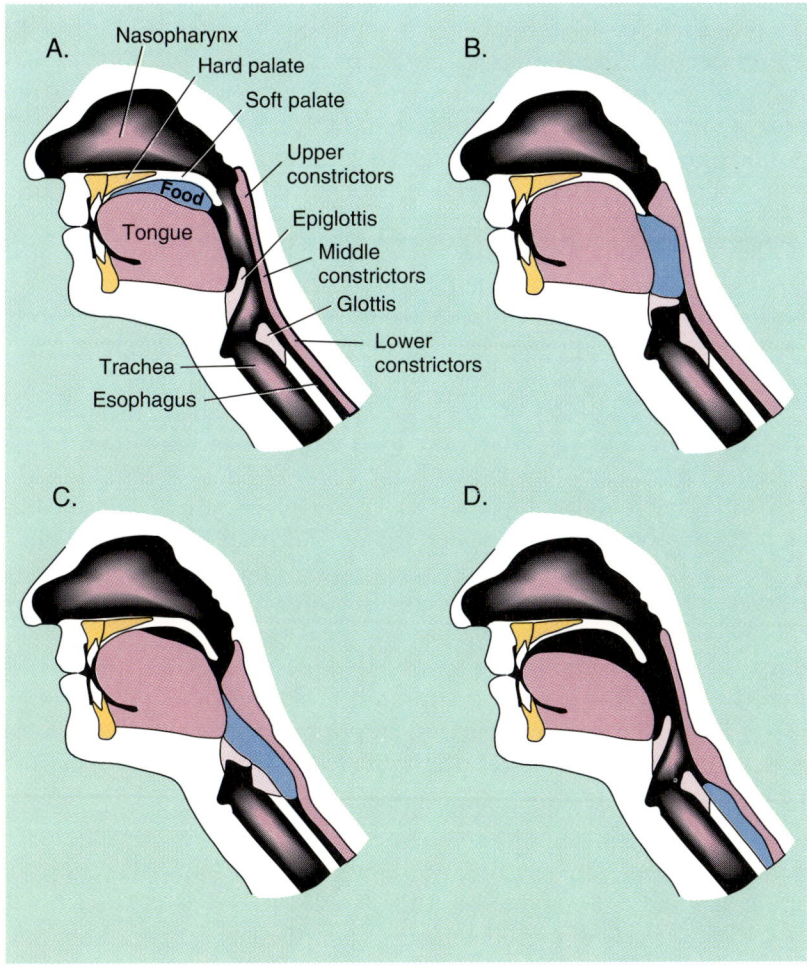

FIGURE 1–4. Mechanical events in the oropharynx during swallowing. *A,* The tongue pushes the chewed food (blue) backward, thereby forcing the soft palate upward toward the upper constrictors of the posterior pharyngeal wall and the epiglottis downward toward the glottis. *B,* The upper constrictor muscles contract and meet the soft palate, thereby sealing the nasopharynx against entry of food. *C,* The glottis is pulled upward to meet the epiglottis, thereby sealing the trachea against entry of food. *D,* The sequential peristaltic contractions of the upper, middle, and lower pharyngeal constrictor muscles have pushed the food into the esophagus as the upper esophageal sphincter (UES) relaxes.

posterior oropharyngeal wall, it triggers sequential peristaltic contractions of the superior, middle, and inferior constrictor (pharyngeal) muscles, which constrict behind the bolus and relax in front of it. This creates a propulsive peristaltic wave, which forces the bolus into the lower pharynx. Simultaneously, the cricopharyngeus muscle (upper esophageal sphincter) relaxes, and the bolus enters the esophagus, after which the upper esophageal sphincter (UES) closes behind it. The peristaltic wave, which started in the pharynx, continues into the esophagus. The foregoing events of oropharyngeal swallowing take 1 sec to occur.

Esophagus

The esophagus in the adult human is about 20 cm long. At rest, pressure inside the body of the esophagus corresponds to intrathoracic pressure (+5 to −5 mm Hg, depending on respiration). However, pressure at the UES may be as high as 100 mm Hg, and pressure at the lower esophageal sphincter (LES) may reach 50 mm Hg. These high sphincteric pressures in the resting esophagus impede air from entering the proximal end of the organ and resist the reflux of acidic gastric juice into the lower end of the esophagus. Peristaltic waves in the esophagus travel with a velocity of 2 cm/sec, pushing food in front of the waves. Solid food takes about 10 sec to move the length of the organ, whereas liquids are propelled from the UES to the LES in 1 or 2 sec.

Within 2 sec of swallowing, the LES relaxes to allow passage of the food into the stomach (Fig. 1–5), and the LES pressure remains low for 6 to 8 sec. Simultaneously, the upper part of the stomach relaxes to receive the new load of food. This mechanical accommodation to the swallowed food by the upper stomach is called "receptive relaxation," and it allows acceptance of large volumes of food with little increase in intraluminal pressure. Thus, ingestion of a large meal might add 1 liter of liquid and solid food to the upper stomach, but result in only a 10–mm Hg increase in pressure. Rapid sizeable increases in stomach pressure would be very uncomfortable and could provoke vomiting. The mechanical events occurring during the esophageal and upper gastric portions of swallowing can be tracked by measuring pressure changes caused by contractions and relaxations prompted by peristalsis and receptive relaxation (see Fig. 1–5).

The process of swallowing food is coordinated primarily by the nervous system (Fig. 1–6). Neural control involves an integrative unit in the medulla, the swallowing center, which receives input from the oropharynx, esophagus, and upper stomach via vagal afferent fibers. The swallowing center also coordinates sequential activities of the following:

1. The respiratory and speech centers, to prevent aspiration of food into the trachea during the oropharyngeal phase of swallowing.
2. The nucleus ambiguous, to initiate and sustain peristaltic contraction of posterior pharyngeal muscles and relaxation of the UES.
3. The dorsal motor nucleus, to initiate and sustain esophageal peristalsis and relax the LES and the upper stomach.

The neural impulses generated by these medullary centers are relayed initially to the vagal nuclei. Vagal efferent fibers then send impulses to the oropharyngeal and upper esophageal striated muscle or to the smooth muscle via the esophageal and gastric portions of the enteric nervous system (Fig. 1–7). Thus, brain stem injury can disrupt swallowing at multiple levels.

The enteric nervous system directly controls swallowing through its innervation of the distal esophageal and proximal gastric smooth muscle. Nerves in the myenteric and

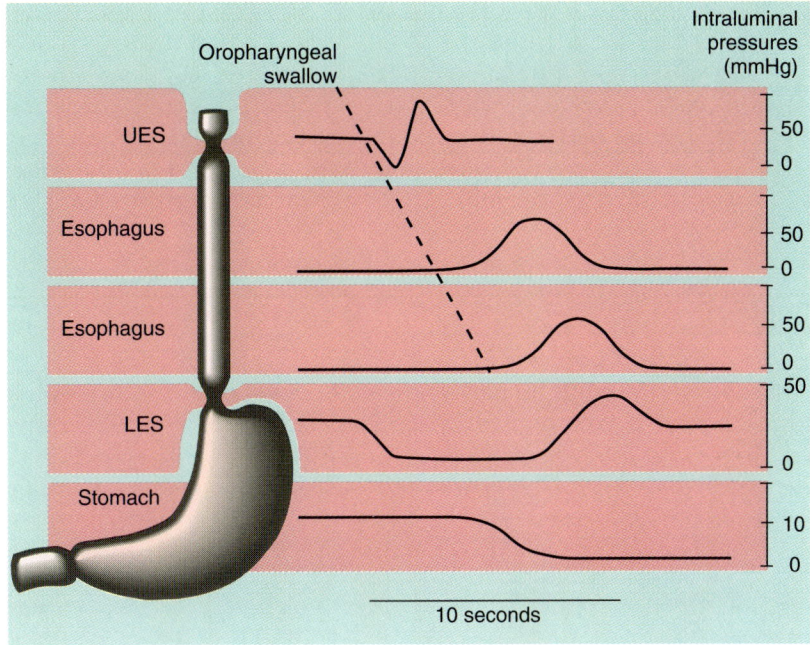

FIGURE 1–5. Swallowing causes sequential contraction in the body of the esophagus and relaxation of the lower esophageal sphincter (LES) and upper stomach. As the swallow commences, the UES relaxes and then contracts. As the peristaltic wave moves along the length of the esophagus, there is a transient increase in pressure at each point where the contraction occurs. However, when the wave reaches the LES, both the LES and the upper stomach relax to receive the bolus of food.

submucosal plexuses are geared to send impulses to near and distant parts of the enteric nervous system (see Fig. 1–7), thereby sustaining peristaltic activity and relaxing the LES after swallowing is initiated. The enteric nervous system is also activated by food stretching the walls of the esophagus. Hence, esophageal peristalsis can occur even after bilateral vagotomy high in the chest. The vagal nerves relax the UES and LES directly. The vagi stimulate the myenteric plexus to initiate peristalsis and to relax the LES. The hormone gastrin increases the tone of the LES, whereas cholecystokinin (CCK) relaxes the LES.

Peptic esophagitis is caused by a failure of the LES to close tightly and function as a barrier against the return of gastric contents. There is reflux of gastric acid into the esophagus, which causes erosion and bleeding of the lower esophageal mucosa. The resulting symptoms include heartburn, indigestion, and a sour taste in the mouth. Esophagitis can cause pain that can be confused with cardiac pain in older patients. It is aggravated by coffee, citrus juice, ethanol, and cigarette smoking.

Stomach

The major functions of the human stomach are to store food and liquid temporarily, to solubilize nutrients, to reduce food particle size, to initiate digestion of food (with salivary and gastric enzymes), and to slowly empty the partly digested contents into the duodenum. The upper portion of the stomach usually lacks peristaltic activity and main-

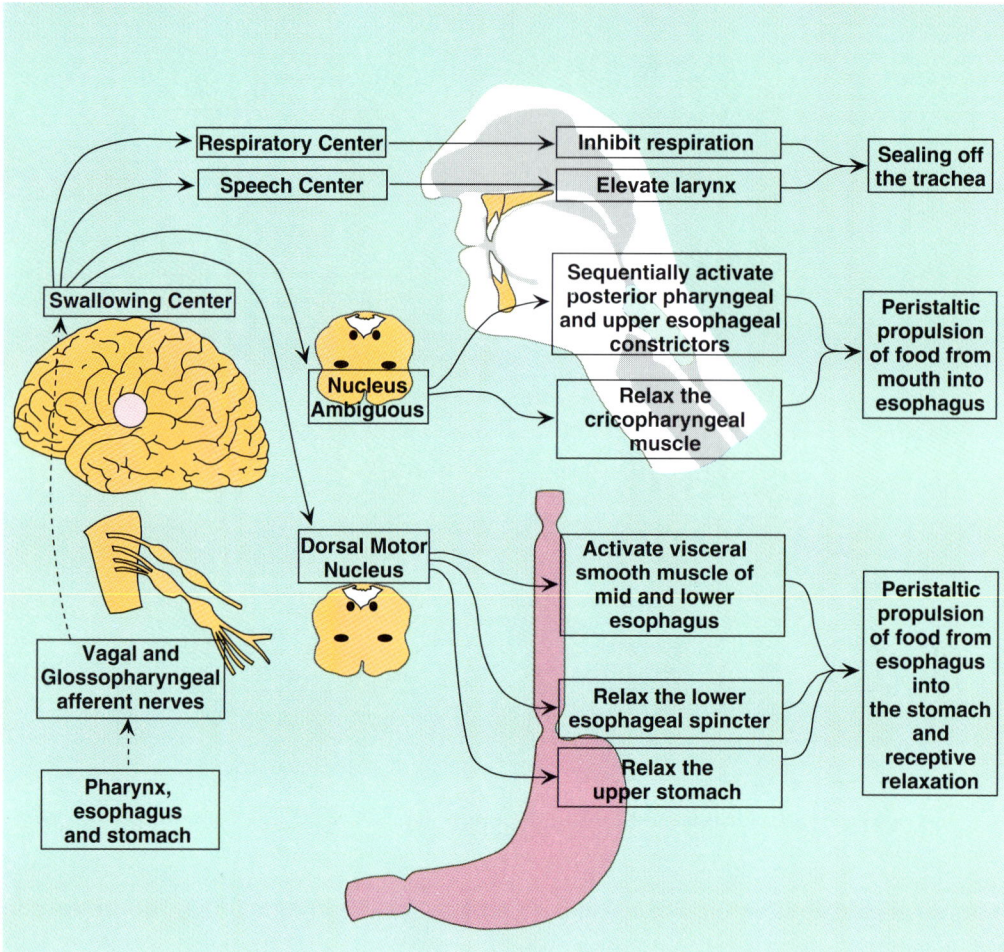

FIGURE 1-6. The swallowing of food and its movement through the pharynx and esophagus and into the stomach requires CNS coordination by the swallowing center. The swallowing center coordinates inhibition of respiratory and speech centers and stimulation of the nucleus ambiguus and the dorsal motor nucleus. These neural interactions permit tracheal closure, pharyngeal peristalsis, opening of the UES, esophageal peristalsis, and opening of the LES. The swallowing center receives information about the progress of the swallow in the pharynx, esophagus, and upper stomach via afferent fibers in the cranial nerves IX and X.

tains a low resting pressure but has a high compliance. Food tends to accumulate in the upper stomach when a large meal is consumed, but this causes little pressure change (i.e., receptive relaxation). As the contents of the stomach are emptied, the upper part of the organ contracts, again with little change in pressure.

The lower part of the stomach displays peristaltic movement, which mixes the food with gastric juice and propels the food and liquid toward the pylorus (Fig. 1–8). The peristaltic waves begin about halfway down the greater curvature and move toward the pylorus. As the wave approaches the pylorus, it increases in both force and velocity. In adults, the duration of a wave at any point on the stomach wall is about 10 sec, and there are typically three peristaltic waves per minute. The wave pushes food and fluid contained in the lumen of the stomach toward the pyloric channel, but the wave moves faster than the gastric contents. Consequently, the wave reaches the pyloric channel before the contents

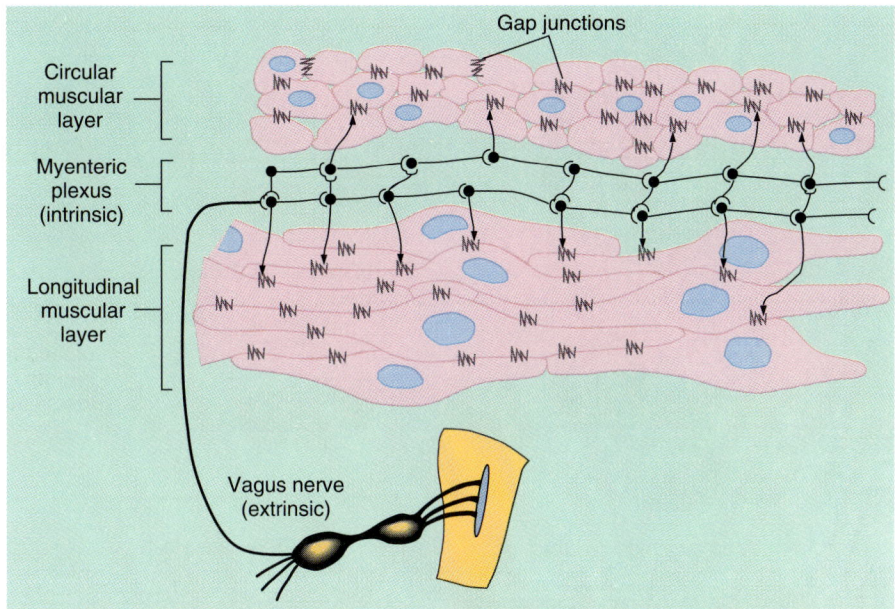

FIGURE 1–7. Esophageal muscle cells are controlled by extrinsic and intrinsic nerves, yet not every muscle cell is innervated. The extrinsic, efferent vagal fibers innervate the intrinsic neurons of the myenteric plexus, located between the circular and longitudinal layers of esophageal smooth muscle cells. The intrinsic nerves innervate some, but not all, of the muscle cells, which in turn are able to excite neighboring cells via their common gap junctions.

and contracts the channel so that only a small part of the moving gastric fluid is actually propelled into the duodenum. Most of the content is squeezed back into the main part of the gastric lumen, a phenomenon called "retropulsion" (see Fig. 1–8). Repeated retropulsive contractions thoroughly mix the food and fluid in the gastric lumen, reducing swallowed solid food to very small size. Particles finally emptied by the stomach into the duodenum are about 1 mm in diameter. Retropulsion also facilitates continued digestion of food in the stomach. After an average mixed meal containing solid food with lipid and fluid totalling 500 ml in volume, coupled with the secretion of another 500 ml of gastric juice and swallowed saliva, 2 hr may elapse before the stomach is emptied. During this time, more than 300 peristaltic waves will have been generated. Retropulsion is one of the mechanisms responsible for the slow rate of gastric emptying.

Halfway down the greater curvature of the stomach, there is also an area of highest excitability or most rapid depolarization known as the "pacemaker." The pacemaker sets the rate of peristaltic contractions, which start at the site and move toward the pyloric sphincter. The pacemaker cells elicit two types of electrical activity—namely, slow waves and spike potentials. Slow waves are cyclic depolarizations of smooth muscle with a frequency of three to five per minute. Spike potentials are periodic fast waves of depolarization that are superimposed on a slow wave after the latter has started. However, the electrical activity only initiates mechanical contractions of the gastric musculature if the slow wave exceeds a threshold value of 5 mV (Fig. 1–9). Spike potentials on slow waves whose amplitude exceeds threshold are always followed by a muscle contraction. Some slow waves do not reach threshold value and hence do not initiate peristaltic waves. Like the peristaltic waves, the slow waves migrate toward the pylorus. Therefore, the peristaltic

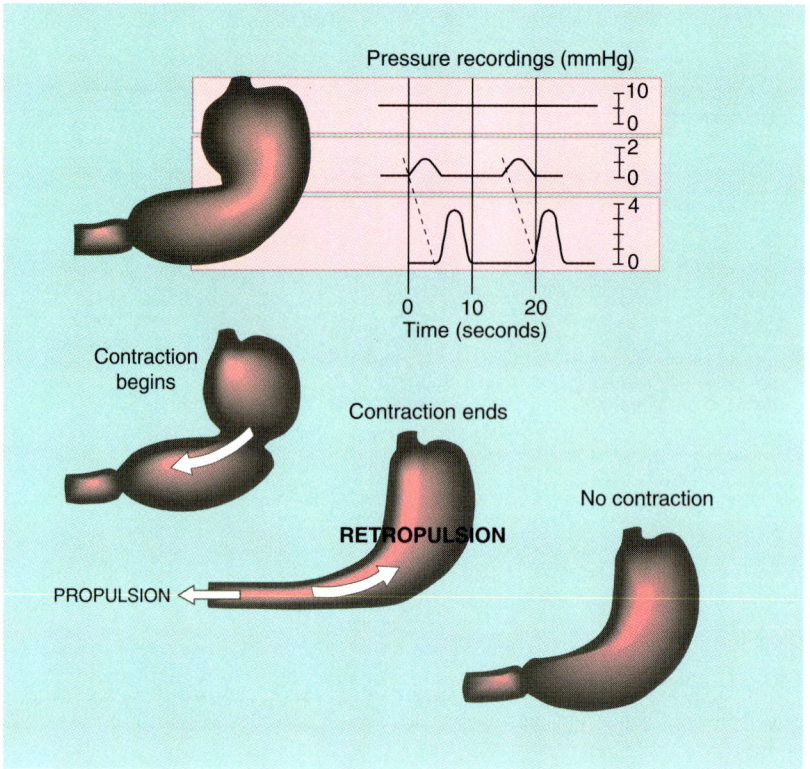

FIGURE 1–8. A contraction of the lower stomach propels only a small volume of chyme into the duodenum. Intraluminal pressure recordings in the upper stomach show a small but steady pressure without peristaltic contractions. The mid and lower portions of the stomach exhibit peristaltic activity, characterized by transient waves of contraction that begin at the mid portion of the greater curvature and progress to the pyloric channel. The movement of chyme toward or away from the small intestine is depicted by the open arrows. The peristaltic wave moves faster than the chyme and reaches the pylorus first, thereby causing a contraction of the pyloric channel. Hence, when the contraction ends, most of the moving chyme is turned back from the pylorus to the stomach (retropulsion). Only a small portion of the chyme is pushed into the duodenum (propulsion).

wave frequency, the direction taken by these waves, and the contractile velocity all depend on the slow waves of muscle depolarization. Furthermore, the greater the electrical amplitude of a slow wave that has exceeded threshold, the greater the force generated by the subsequent peristaltic wave.

Both the regularity and the direction of slow waves across the stomach wall are disorganized by surgical interruption of the vagus nerves. Hence, impaired gastric emptying of solids with resultant bezoar formation is a consequence of bilateral vagotomy at the level of the diaphragm. Greater gastrin release, however, increases the frequency of slow waves. Vagal nerve stimulation increases the amplitude and the frequency of both slow waves and the resulting peristaltic contractions (Fig. 1–10). Therefore, both vagal stimulation and gastrin enhance the emptying of the stomach.

At the pyloric sphincter there are three sets of contracting muscle, all of which influence emptying of the stomach in a different way. The smooth muscle wall of the lower

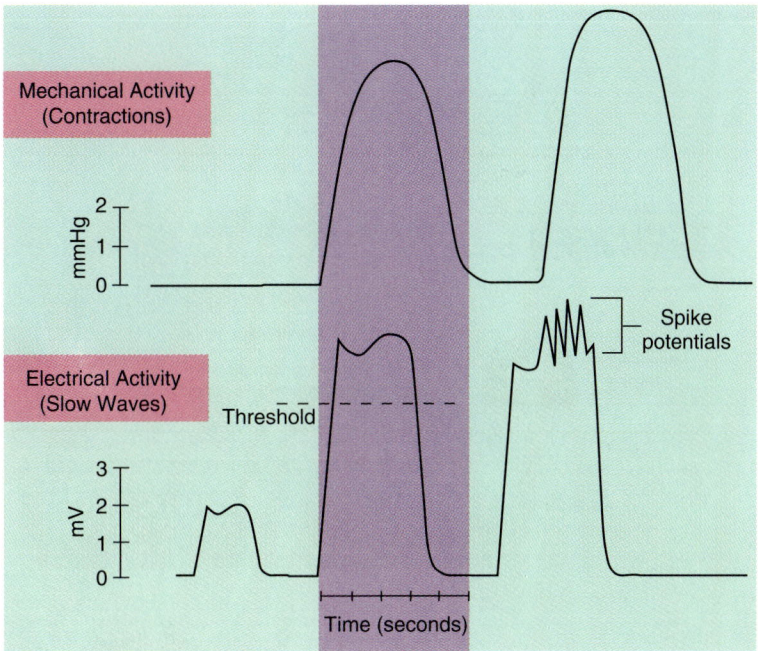

FIGURE 1–9. Mechanical contractions depend on slow waves that exceed a threshold value and on spike potentials. When the peak amplitude of a slow wave is below threshold (about 5 mV), there is no subsequent contraction of the gastric muscle. When the slow wave exceeds threshold, there is usually a peristaltic contraction of the muscle (measured in mm Hg of intraluminal pressure). Frequently, there are rapid, recurrent, small depolarizations (spike potentials) that are superimposed on those slow waves that have exceeded threshold. Spike potentials are always followed by a mechanical contraction of gastric smooth muscle.

stomach contracts at a maximal rate of four peristaltic waves per minute. This motor activity tends to propel the gastric contents into the duodenum, albeit slowly. The smooth muscle walls of the duodenum contract about 12 times per minute. However, many of these contractions reflect only the contractile activity of the circular smooth muscle layer in the duodenal wall, are not propulsive, and are known as "rhythmic segmentation." Rhythmic segmentation acts to resist gastric emptying of chyme into the duodenum. At the interface between the stomach and duodenum is the pyloric sphincter, a muscle thickening that can contract partially to increase wall tension or contract more forcefully to narrow the pyloric channel. In either case, contractions of the pyloric sphincter oppose gastric emptying of chyme into the duodenum.

Another factor that influences gastric emptying is the composition of the material being emptied. Water is emptied the most rapidly (i.e., in a few minutes). Solid food resides in the stomach for many minutes or even hours, because its size must be reduced by repeated retropulsion and because the chemical or physical composition of the food may evoke neuroendocrine mechanisms that inhibit gastric emptying. Three major variables in the quality of gastric contents slow gastric emptying: increased acidity, lipid content, and osmolality. These variables act via direct contact with the duodenal mucosa to stimulate release of the hormones secretin, CCK, and gastric inhibitory peptide (GIP) and to initiate a local neural reflex. The consequences of activating these neurohumoral mech-

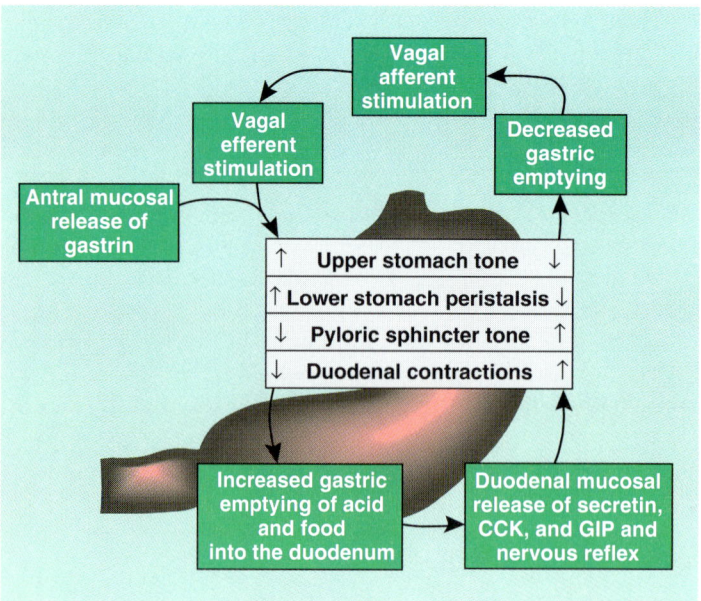

FIGURE 1–10. Gastric emptying waxes and wanes because of opposing mechanisms. Emptying of the stomach is facilitated by increased vagal nerve activity and gastrin release, which increase upper gastric pressure and peristalsis of the lower stomach while decreasing pyloric sphincter tone and duodenal contractions. As the stomach empties its gastric juice and partly digested food, peptide hormones released from the duodenal mucosa and a nervous reflex decrease upper gastric tone and inhibit lower gastric peristaltic activity while increasing both pyloric sphincteric pressure and duodenal contractions. Thus, increased gastric emptying acts to inhibit subsequent emptying, and decreased gastric emptying acts to stimulate subsequent gastric emptying. GIP = Gastric inhibitory peptide.

anisms are relaxation of the upper stomach, inhibition of lower stomach peristaltic activity, an increase in pyloric sphincter motor activity, and stimulation of duodenal rhythmic segmentation. These events inhibit gastric emptying for a time (see Fig. 1–10).

The stomach containing ingested solid and liquid food and gastric secretions transmits its message about the need for emptying via vagal afferent nerves to the medulla and then to the hypothalamus. A stimulatory relay is elicited from the hypothalamus, which activates vagal nuclei in the medulla to transmit impulses via vagal efferent nerves to the stomach and duodenum. The results are gastrin release, upper gastric smooth muscle activation, stimulation of lower gastric peristalsis, pyloric sphincter relaxation, and inhibition of duodenal rhythmic segmentation. This combination of events is conducive to the emptying of gastric contents into the duodenum, and the cycle of stimulation followed by inhibition of gastric emptying is under way (see Fig. 1–10).

After gastric digestion of some food and emptying of the digested, dissolved, and disintegrated nutrients (collectively known as chyme) into the duodenum, some non-nutrient material still remains in the stomach. This material includes indigestible and insoluble vegetable fiber, mostly cellulose. These large particles are emptied by an abrupt and transient burst of powerful peristaltic contractions that begin in the upper stomach and sweep down the entire organ, propelling the remaining gastric content into the duodenum and then down the length of the small intestine. This infrequent activity is called the "migrating motor complex" (MMC). The MMC occurs after a meal and after completion of gastric emptying. Following the MMC, the stomach is in a quiescent state for 1 to 2 hr before peristaltic activity resumes.

Vomiting is most often a nonpathological event, infrequent, and short lived. However, protracted or frequent vomiting may be indicative of serious pathology. Just before vomiting, there is usually a sense that vomiting is impending, a feeling known as "nausea," and there is a diffuse discharge of sympathetic and parasympathetic nerves. Careful physical observation of a patient about to vomit reveals sympathetic responses such as pallor, sweating, cold skin, and increased cardiac and respiratory rates. Occult parasympathetic responses include increased salivation, enhanced motor activity in the stomach and esophagus, and relaxation of the LES and UES. The individual about to vomit takes a deep breath, closes the glottis, contracts the abdominal muscles, and squeezes the stomach between the diaphragm and the abdominal muscles, thereby abruptly emptying the stomach. The gastric content is rapidly propelled up the esophagus, past the relaxed LES and UES, and out of the mouth.

Small Intestine

Small intestinal motility varies and causes mixing of nutrients and digestive enzymes; increased mucosal surface exposure to digested nutrients, which facilitates nutrient absorption; and aboral propulsion of undigested materials. A comparison of propulsive movements (peristalsis) and mixing contractions (rhythmic segmentation) is shown in Figure 1–11.

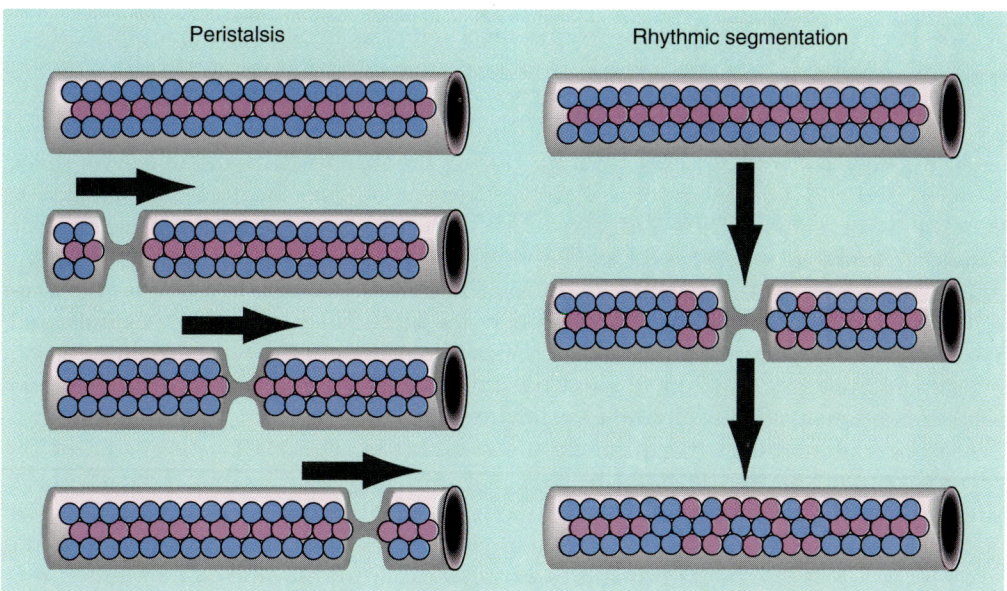

FIGURE 1–11. Peristalsis propels chyme, and rhythmic segmentation mixes chyme. Peristalsis appears as a propagated wave of contraction that pushes the chyme aborally in front of the moving wave. Rhythmic segmentation is the result of contractions and relaxations of only the circular muscle layer. Hence, the contractions are not propagated and do not propel the chyme. However, rhythmic segmentation does serve to mix and redistribute the components of chyme, thereby aiding both digestion and absorption of nutrients.

Smooth muscle in the muscularis of the small intestine is organized into an inner, thicker, circular muscle layer and an outer, thinner, longitudinal muscle layer. Both layers are thicker in the proximal half of the organ than in the ileum.

The neural elements of the small intestine consist of intrinsic and extrinsic nerves that are in communication with one another. Intrinsic nerves of the enteric nervous system are located mainly in the myenteric and submucosal plexuses. The enteric nervous system of the small intestine, colon, esophagus, and stomach is a vast collection of neurons, equal in number to the population of nerves in the spinal cord. Not unexpectedly, there are a variety of nerve types in the myenteric and submucosal plexuses, with an even greater variety of neurotransmitters, most of which affect motility. In addition to acetylcholine and catecholamines, other important transmitters in the enteric nervous system include neuropeptides (e.g., substance P, vasoactive intestinal peptide (VIP), neuropeptide Y, calcitonin gene-related peptide, CCK, enkephalins, tachykinins, bradykinin, and somatostatin), amines (e.g., histamine, glutamine, and 5-hydroxytryptamine), nitric oxide, gamma-aminobutyrate, and purines (e.g., adenosine and ATP).

Many of these neurotransmitters are also produced by enterochromaffin cells, mast cells, endothelial cells, and even parenchymal cells of the mucosa. Some of these neurocrine substances may also act as either endocrine substances (e.g., blood-borne hormones such as CCK) or paracrine substances (e.g., histamine), which are released into the interstitium, where they diffuse to cell surface receptors. Visceral smooth muscle cells are often the target of these agents. Extrinsic nerves include the vagal, parasympathetic, preganglionic nerves, whose transmitters include acetylcholine, VIP, and ATP, and the splanchnic, sympathetic, postganglionic nerves, whose transmitters include norepinephrine, ATP, and neuropeptide Y.

When the small intestine is at rest and no contractions are occurring, the pressure in the lumen is equal to intraabdominal pressure (i.e., +10 to −10 mm Hg, but usually near 0 mm Hg). Most contractions of the small intestine involve less than 5 cm of the length of the organ, last for about 5 sec, and are separated from the next contraction by about 5 sec.

Between meals, the small bowel exhibits an overall interdigestive pattern of protracted inactivity followed by quite active periods. During the inactive state, there are no spikes of electrical depolarization and no muscular contractions. This inaction is terminated by the onset of occasional spikes and contractions, which accelerate into frequent depolarizations and forceful contractions. During this period of intense motor activity, there are contractile complexes that start in the stomach and proximal small intestine and migrate along the bowel to the ileocecal junction where the MMC fades. As one MMC disappears, another MMC starts in the stomach and upper gut. The MMC has a velocity of about 6 cm/min and requires 1 to 2 hr to move from the stomach to the cecum. The MMC propels small intestinal contents into the cecum, thereby reducing the accumulation of undigested materials and microorganisms in the small bowel. The MMC is triggered by the peptide motilin, which is released by proximal small intestinal enterochromaffin cells. MMC activity is also stimulated by other gastrointestinal paracrine substances (e.g., somatostatin and pancreatic polypeptide), neuropeptide transmitters (e.g., substance P and enkephalins). MMC activity is brought to a halt by eating and by hormones released during feeding and digestion of food (e.g., CCK, gastrin, and insulin). With feeding, the interdigestive pattern of long inactive periods alternating with MMC periods is replaced. For several hours the less regular digestive phase of small intestinal motor activity dominates.

In people who have eaten recently, peristaltic activity is more orderly. Motility consists of a few contractions following one another, with fixed intervals between them. The train of contractions is followed by periods of no contractions. These inactive periods last 5, 10 or 15 sec.

Slow waves of muscle depolarization occur in the small intestine; the amplitude of their depolarizations is about 10 mV. There are a maximum of 12 slow waves per min in the duodenum, where the pacemaker is located near the entry point of the common bile duct. The electrical firing frequency decreases gradually along the small intestine to the distal ileum, where the frequency of depolarizations is only eight per min. When spike potentials are superimposed on the slow wave depolarization phase, a mechanical contraction of the small intestine ensues. However, spike potentials do not occur on all slow waves. Therefore, the maximum mechanical contractile rate anywhere in the small bowel cannot exceed the slow wave frequency of that gut segment. Accordingly, on average, there is one slow wave every 5 sec and a maximum of one contraction every 5 sec. Contractions may also occur every 10 or 15 sec, depending on the prevalence of slow waves containing spike potentials. The velocity of the peristaltic waves moving down the length of the small intestine equals that of the slow waves moving through the smooth muscle mass.

Peristaltic activity in the small intestine can be inhibited by neurotoxic agents that act on the enteric nervous system, by vagotomy, by distention of nearby gut, and by emotional state (epinephrine inhibits peristalsis). Stimulation of peristalsis occurs with increased vagal activity and in response to hormones (e.g., gastrin, CCK, and insulin) and paracrine agents (e.g., 5-hydroxytryptamine and prostaglandins). Several neurotransmitters, paracrine substances, and the hormone motilin activate MMC.

Rhythmic segmentation consists of transient, nonpropulsive, mechanical contractions of circular muscle (see Fig. 1–11). These contractions mix chyme with digestive enzymes and increase the mucosal surface area available for absorption of nutrients. Rhythmic segmentation is observed everywhere in the small bowel and in the colon.

In addition, both the villi and the folds of Kerckring contain visceral smooth muscle. Its contractions and relaxations cause the villi and the folds to undulate. These movements also mix the chyme and expose more surface area for absorption of nutrients.

Chyme propelled into the distal ileum distends that part of the small intestine and initiates a reflex in the enteric nervous system, which causes the ileocecal junction to relax (Fig. 1–12). The peristaltic wave then squirts the chyme into the cecum, thereby distending the proximal colon, which reflexly causes the ileocecal junction to contract and prevent the reflux of chyme back into the ileum. The increase in ileal peristalsis and the opening of the junction occur mainly during the postprandial period and appear to be stimulated by increasing plasma concentrations of gastrin and CCK combined with a neural reflex.

Colon

The major functions of the human colon include storing the liquid chyme from the ileum, absorbing water and salt from the chyme, permitting bacterial action, and excreting residual material, which at this point has become semisolid. Storage of the chyme occupies several days, during which time absorption of fluid and electrolytes occurs. Excretion of the semisolid residual feces occupies a matter of a few minutes.

The colon is a 75-cm-long tube with a sacculated appearance and three strips of longitudinal muscle running most of the length of the organ. The saccules, termed "haustrae," are formed because of the limiting length of the longitudinal muscle strips, called "taenia coli." The lack of a continuous layer of longitudinal smooth muscle surrounding

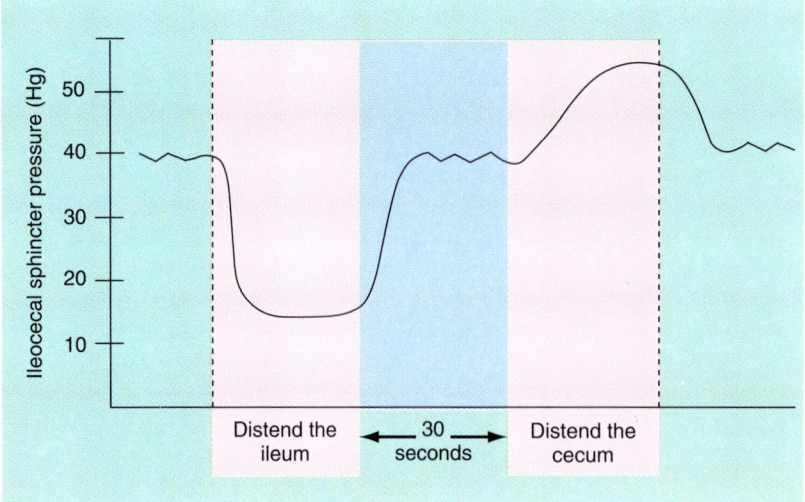

FIGURE 1–12. The ileocecal sphincter relaxes when the ileum is distended and contracts when the cecum is distended. By analogy, when a peristaltic wave propels chyme into the distal ileum, that part of the small intestine is distended, and a reflex neural mechanism relaxes the ileocecal sphincter, permitting propulsion of chyme from the ileum into the cecum. The cecum is distended at this point and triggers a different reflex, which causes the sphincteric pressure to increase greatly; this prevents any retropulsion of cecal contents into the ileum as the distended cecum contracts.

the colon is responsible for the lack of the usual peristaltic waves in most of the colon. Nevertheless, there are propulsive and retropulsive movements in the colon. Thus, in the ascending colon, the contents are pushed toward the cecum by retrograde annular contractions. These retropulsive movements cause retention of liquid chyme, allowing absorption of water and electrolytes and conversion of luminal contents into semisolid feces. In the transverse colon, the major activity is rhythmic segmentation, which mixes fecal contents. In the sigmoid colon, peristaltic contractions propel feces into the rectum. Peristalsis also takes place in the rectum, which contains a continuous layer of longitudinal muscle. In the rectal wall, distal to the internal anal sphincter, thick striated muscle forms the external anal sphincter. The external anal sphincter can be relaxed or contracted voluntarily.

The proximal two thirds of the colon is innervated by the vagus nerves, whereas the pelvic preganglionic parasympathetic nerves supply the descending and sigmoid portions of the colon and most of the rectum. The postganglionic sympathetic nerves emerge from the superior mesenteric ganglion to innervate the proximal two thirds of the colon. The inferior mesenteric ganglion supplies sympathetic fibers to the rest of the organ as far as the distal rectum. The hypogastric ganglion sends sympathetic neurons to reach the terminal part of the rectum and anal canal. The external anal sphincter, which is comprised of striated muscle, is innervated by the somatic pudendal nerves. Parasympathetic nerves activate colonic motility, both directly and via synapses with the enteric nervous system. Sympathetic nerves inhibit colonic motility and constrict blood vessels to the colon. Most of the enteric nervous system of the colon is located in the myenteric plexus, which is concentrated beneath the taenia coli in much of the organ, and in the submucosal plexus. Enteric neurotransmitters include acetylcholine, neuropeptides, amines, and purines.

The most common motor activity observed in the colon is rhythmic segmentation, which is caused by contraction of the abundant circular muscle. These movements mix the chyme and expose the colonic mucosa to Na^+, Cl^-, and water for absorption. Rhythmic segmentation also prevents propulsion of the chyme to the rectum. These contractions last longer (up to 1 min) than their counterparts in the small intestine and generate higher pressures (up to 50 mm Hg).

Mass movement is the major type of propulsive motility in the colon. When mass movement starts (usually after a meal), a large bolus traverses a long distance of the large bowel fairly fast (Fig. 1–13). Once the feces reach the rectum, peristaltic waves begin again. These waves are fairly rapid and move the fecal bolus deeper into the rectum, where it is stored temporarily. The frequent occurrence of mass movement after meals is suggestive of a gastrocolic reflex; however, patients who have sustained a gastrectomy still exhibit mass movement. Colonic motility appears to be neurally controlled.

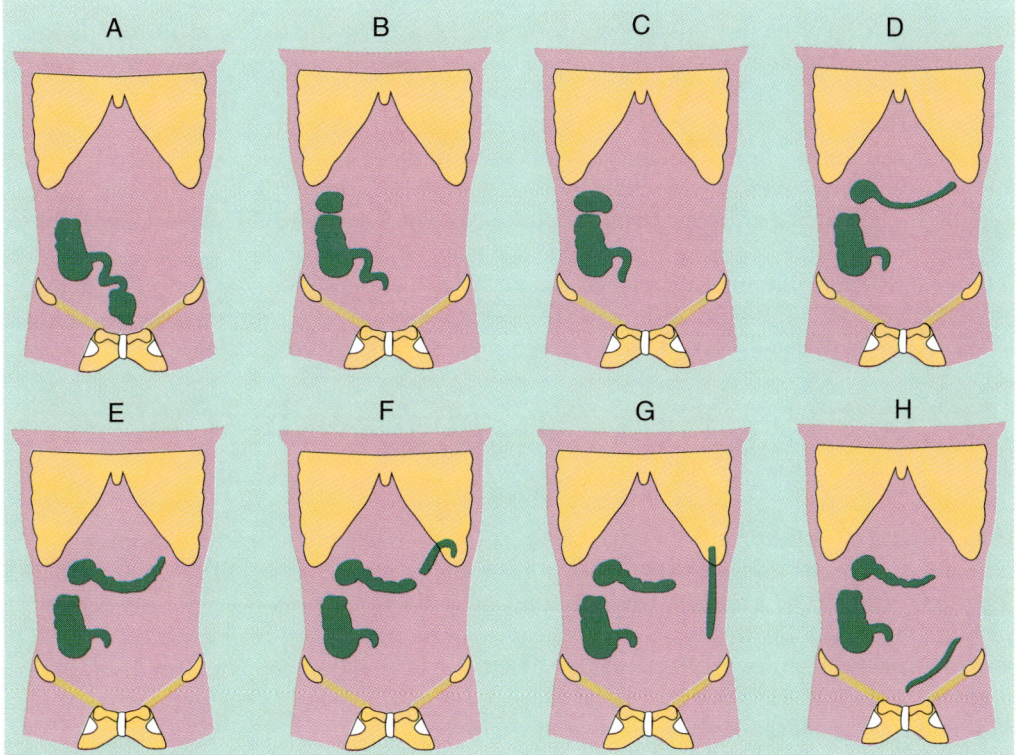

FIGURE 1–13. Mass movement of colonic contents involves moderately rapid propulsion. The patient depicted in the figure swallowed 60 ml radiopaque barium sulfate ($BaSO_4$) solution with breakfast at 7 AM. The results of the first radiograph, obtained at noon, are illustrated in A, where the $BaSO_4$-coated feces are visible in the ileum, cecum, and ascending colon. Then the patient ate lunch. By the end of lunch (B) some of the $BaSO_4$-coated feces had separated from the main mass. As shown in C through E, the separated material was propelled around the hepatic flexure and along the transverse colon. F through H, A portion of the separated feces was pinched off and moved around the splenic flexure, along the descending colon, and into the sigmoid colon. Mass movement (from B to H) occupied about 15 min, during which time the feces were propelled about 75 cm.

Rectum

The two major motor functions of the human rectum are to briefly store fecal material and to participate in its excretion. Feces are stored until it is convenient to defecate. Stored feces stretch the wall of the rectum and initiate a reflex that relaxes the internal anal sphincter. Fecal stretching of the anal canal follows, and the person feels the urge to defecate. Voluntary contraction of the striated muscle of the external anal sphincter inhibits the reflex, causing the rectal wall to relax and the internal anal sphincter to close. At the appropriate time and place, the person voluntarily relaxes the external anal sphincter; this is aided by a sitting or squatting posture. Extra pressure is applied to the outside of the rectum by voluntarily contracting the abdominal muscles and exhaling against a closed glottis, thereby raising pressure in the thoracic and abdominal cavities while lowering the pelvic floor. Thus, pressure is imposed on the rectum from the outside, and fecal material is expelled from the anal canal.

Constipation is a common complaint among Americans, providing the impetus to flourishing businesses that annually market billions of dollars worth of laxatives and breakfast cereals. It is difficult to define constipation, because it is partly subjective. For some people, failure to defecate once each day constitutes constipation and is a cause for alarm. For other people "regularity" is a more casual matter, and such people do not complain about constipation, even after going several days without defecating. Constipation can be considered to exist when a person fails to defecate three times per week, despite eating the usual kinds of food on a regular basis. Constipation involves two changes in colonic function: (1) increased storage capacity of the cecum and ascending and transverse parts of the colon and (2) decreased propulsive capacity of the descending colon and sigmoid. The major factors that diminish the frequency of bowel movements include (1) diets low in insoluble fiber (i.e., nonstarch, complex polysaccharides), (2) diets low in the volume of fluid consumed, and (3) old age. The first two factors are correctable.

CASE REPORTS: CONCLUSION

• Case 1 •

CLINICAL IMPRESSION. Esophageal spasm, either reflux induced or idiopathic. The infrequency of the chest pain makes historical correlation with life events difficult. The lack of objective evidence for reflux on the tests performed does not necessarily exclude the possibility that, in certain circumstances, the patient may experience gastroesophageal reflux precipitating esophageal spasm and chest pain. Similarly, the inability to document spasm during an esophageal motility study does not exclude idiopathic esophageal spasm as a cause of the pain.

At this point, the patient was educated about potential causes of her pain and the exclusion of causes that would threaten her health (e.g., cardiac and pulmonary causes). She was also informed that surgical therapy at this stage might cause more problems than her current symptoms. To completely exclude reflux as a potential source of the pain, the patient was placed on omeprazole (20 mg daily) for 3 months. If the pain continued or worsened, consideration would be given to the use of low-dose tricyclic antidepressants (e.g., trazodone), which have been reported to reduce symptoms in idiopathic esophageal spasm.

With institution of omeprazole, the chest pain stopped. Ultimately the patient and physician elected to stop medication because of the infrequency of symptoms. She has rare attacks that are controlled with an anxiolytic agent taken at the onset of pain.

• Case 2 •

CLINICAL IMPRESSION. Chronic functional constipation. Even when constipation has been lifelong, it is important to perform a thorough evaluation to exclude structural or metabolic causes. In particular, adult Hirschsprung's disease must be considered.

Initial evaluation revealed that serum electrolyte, blood urea nitrogen (BUN), thyroid-stimulating hormone, Mg^{++}, Ca^{++}, and glucose levels were normal. A barium enema demonstrated a redundant colon with no obstructions, diverticulae, or mucosal lesions. Results of sigmoidoscopy were normal. Attempts to get the patient to incorporate more fiber in her diet led to unacceptable bloating and were discontinued by the patient before any change in bowel habit occurred. Defecography and anorectal manometry were performed, and results were within normal limits.

With this information, an extended educational intervention was undertaken to explain the relationship among fiber, bowel habits, and bloating. Different types of fiber (e.g., rice bran, hemicellulose) were incorporated into the diet at very low doses, with a gradual increase as dictated by the patient's tolerance; it was expected that 6 to 12 months might be required to complete the process. One year later the patient was taking a daily fiber supplement, having a tolerable amount of bloating, and experiencing a bowel movement every other day.

CLINICAL OVERVIEW

Case 1: Esophageal Motor Disorder

In the first case report, the prominent symptom of the swallowing disorder was chest pain. However, pain as a manifestation of disordered esophageal motility is infrequent, unpredictable, and not easily elicited during a 24-hr motility assessment, much less during the confines of a 30-min careful esophageal manometry. The problems involved in relating episodic esophageal pain to pressure tracings deprive the physician of a quantifiable evaluation of the pain and make diagnosis difficult. Not surprisingly, at the time of manometric testing, less than 25% of patients with a history of noncardiac chest pain simultaneously manifest both esophageal pain and abnormal motility patterns. Another 25% of patients exhibit an abnormal motility pattern without experiencing pain during the manometric evaluation. The remaining half of such patients demonstrate normal esophageal manometry. The two major causes of esophageal pain that can be identified manometrically are diffuse esophageal spasm and achalasia. In the former disorder, non-peristaltic, high-pressure, prolonged contractions are noted (Fig. 1–14), whereas achalasia involves an abnormally elevated LES resting pressure that does not fully relax during a swallow (Fig. 1–15).

Case 2: Functional Constipation

The most common cause of constipation is dietary inadequacy—namely, a low intake of insoluble fiber and fluid. Constipation is rarely caused by a definable colonic motor disorder. Dietary fiber provides mass for the colonic content and retains fluid, both of which serve to reduce fecal transit time and colonic wall tension during mass movement and defecation. In patients with rectal motor disorders causing constipation, abnormal

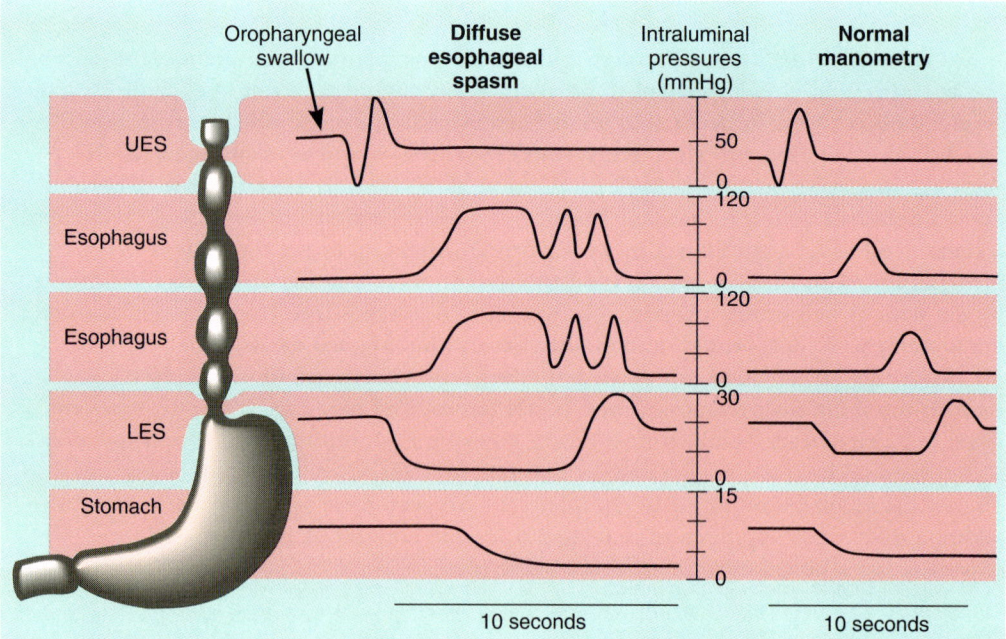

FIGURE 1–14. Manometric findings in the esophagus with diffuse esophageal spasm. The major abnormalities are markedly elevated contraction pressures, protracted periods of contraction, repetitive contractions, and a loss of peristaltic wave progression in the body of the esophagus.

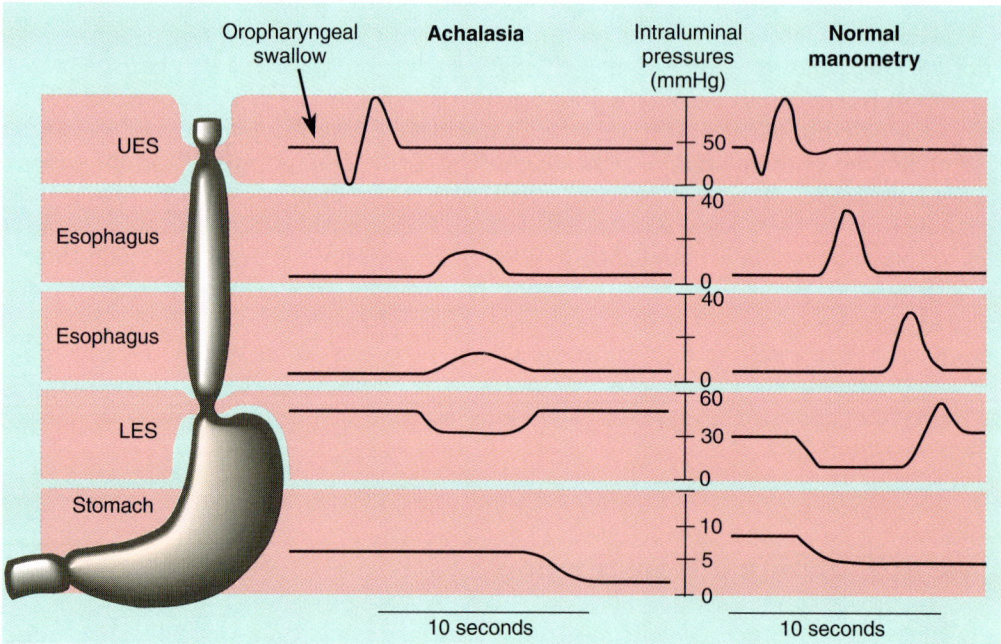

FIGURE 1–15. Manometric findings at different levels of the esophagus during a swallow in a patient with achalasia. Compared with the normal findings shown on the right side of the diagram, the contractions in the esophageal body are feeble and nonperistaltic, and the LES has a high resting pressure that does not fully relax after a swallow.

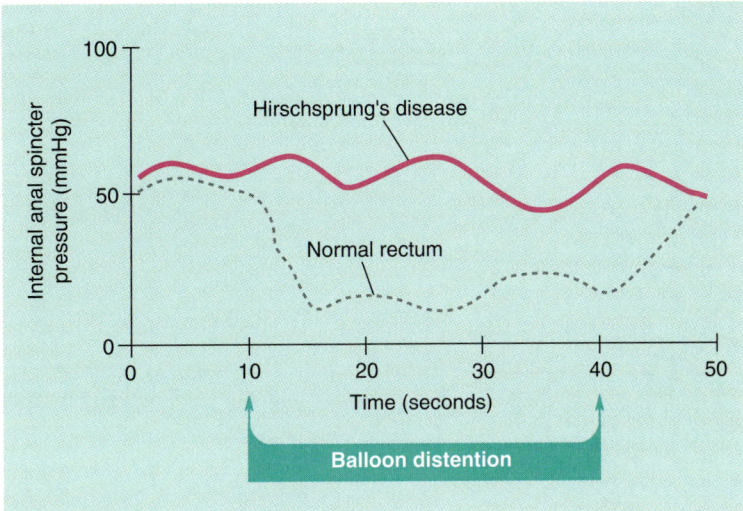

FIGURE 1–16. Anorectal manometry in a normal rectum (dashed line) and in the rectum of a patient with Hirschsprung's disease (solid line). On distention of a small balloon to 60 ml in the upper rectum, the internal anal sphincter normally relaxes. This relaxation does not occur in patients with Hirschsprung's disease.

pressure tracings can be identified during anorectal manometry (Fig. 1–16). For many people, constipation is not perceived as a problem requiring medical attention or self-treatment with laxatives unless they suffer pain or bleeding from enlarged hemorrhoidal veins during defecation. Patients with irritable bowel syndrome, a prevalent colonic motor disorder, may present with constipation as a prominent symptom. It is possible that future technological developments in measuring colonic motility, combined with a better understanding of the pathophysiology, will permit more specific diagnoses of irritable bowel syndrome, as well as functional constipation.

CHAPTER TWO

Gastric Secretion

CASE REPORT: INITIAL INFORMATION

A 54-year-old man was brought to the emergency room by his wife because of nausea, vomiting, and weight loss of 3 weeks duration.

The man had been in his usual state of health until 7 weeks before this time, when he developed burning pain in his epigastrium that did not radiate. The pain was reduced by eating or taking antacids and would wake him from sleep between 2 and 3 AM each night. Gradually the relief provided by eating or antacids diminished. Three weeks before this time he began to vomit. The emesis was composed of undigested food and mucus without blood, was always preceded by nausea, and typically occurred 2 to 4 hr after eating. In the 3 days before coming to the emergency room, the patient became dizzy while arising from a supine position. He had lost 5 kg during the preceding 7 weeks.

The patient had had similar epigastric pain episodically over the preceding 12 years. Four years previously, an upper gastrointestinal series showed an ulcer in the duodenal bulb. Treatment with cimetidine (800 mg at bedtime for 6 weeks) resolved the pain, but it recurred 3 months later. He had seen a physician subsequently until the present illness. No history of hematemesis or melena was noted.

The patient had adult-onset diabetes that was managed with oral hypoglycemic agents and diet. Depression over a previous divorce had led to his being placed on amitriptyline (50 mg hs) 2 years ago. He was a plant supervisor and under stress at work, smoked one pack of cigarettes every day, and only rarely drank alcohol or caffeinated beverages.

The patient's father had had chronic ulcer disease that led to a vagotomy and an antrectomy at age 42, and his brother had had an ulcer treated medically.

On physical examination, his resting pulse of 90 beats/min when supine rose to 120 beats/min in the upright position, and the respective blood pressures changed from 110/80 to 100/60 mm Hg. The examination was normal except for epigastric tenderness without rebound or guarding. A succussion splash was audible. The stool was brown and negative for occult blood. There were no stigmata of chronic liver disease.

LABORATORY FINDINGS. Hematocrit (Hct) = 49%; white blood cell (WBC) count = 12,500 with a normal differential; blood urea nitrogen (BUN) = 68 mg/dl; creatinine = 1.2 mg/dl; Na^+ = 134 mmol/L; K^+ = 2.8 mmol/L; Cl^- = 90 mmol/L; CO_2 = 39 mm Hg; arterial blood gas analysis = normal except for a pH of 7.56; urinalysis = normal except for 2+ glucose; serum glucose = 310 mg/dl; calcium and amylase values normal; albumin = 3.4 gm/dl. A nasogastric tube was placed in the stomach, and 1300 ml of fluid was aspirated. An intravenous infusion was started, the patient was admitted to the hospital, and a gastroenterology consult was ordered.

PHYSIOLOGY

This chapter describes the physiology of the secretory processes in the stomach, including the mechanisms involved in secreting the inorganic and organic components of the gastric juice and the control of gastric secretion. The stomach is a medically important structure because of the widespread, serious illnesses associated with the organ and its secretory functions (e.g., peptic ulcers, gastritis, esophagitis, pernicious anemia, and stomach cancer.

Anatomical Considerations

The gross anatomical regions of the stomach are the fundus, corpus, and antrum (Fig. 2–1). The mucosal surface is divided according to the type of gland—namely, the oxyntic gland area, which secretes acid, and the pyloric gland area, which does not. The most important cell types in these glandular areas are mucous and peptic cells, which are found in both glandular areas; oxyntic (or parietal) cells, which occur only in the oxyntic gland area; and endocrine cells, which are scattered throughout both glandular areas. Most of the mucosal surface of the stomach is occupied by the oxyntic gland area (see Fig. 2–1).

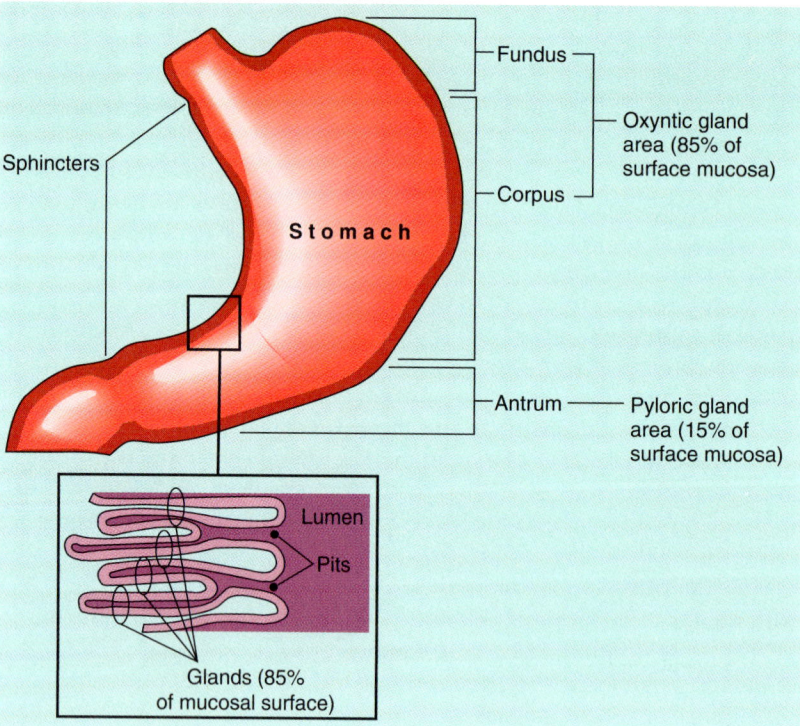

FIGURE 2–1. Eighty-five percent of gastric mucosal surface lines the fundus and corpus, and 85% of total mucosal surface lines the glands in any part of the stomach wall. Most of the gross mucosal surface visible to the unaided eye covers the fundus and corpus, but most of the actual mucosal surface is not visible to the unaided eye, because it lines the glands.

The wall of the stomach consists of four tissues: the mucosa, submucosa, muscularis, and serosa. The mucosal surface lines the gastric lumen and is dotted by the gastric pits, which are the openings of the gastric glands. The mucosal surface extends into and lines the glands. The lining of the glands constitutes most of the functional surface of the gastric mucosa.

The oxyntic gland has three parts: the pit, the neck, and the glandular portion (Fig. 2–2). The pit is lined by mucous surface cells, which secrete mucus and HCO_3^-. The neck contains mucous neck cells, which are the germinal cells of all other glandular cell types. These germinal cells migrate either superficially toward the pit or more deeply into the glands. The glandular portion of the oxyntic gland area contains oxyntic cells, which secrete hydrochloric acid (HCl) and the intrinsic factor (IF). Located deeper in the oxyntic glands are the peptic cells, which secrete pepsinogen. The oxyntic glands also contain mucous cells, as well as endocrine cells that secrete peptides locally and into the blood. In the actively secreting stomach (e.g., at mealtime), the oxyntic cells are responsible for secreting nearly all of the gastric juice (Fig. 2–3).

Oxyntic cells make up one third of the cells of the oxyntic gland area. Peptic and mucous cells each make up one fourth of the cells of the gland. Other important cell types found in the mucosa include connective tissue cells, mast cells, visceral muscle cells, nerve cells, vascular muscle cells, and endothelial cells.

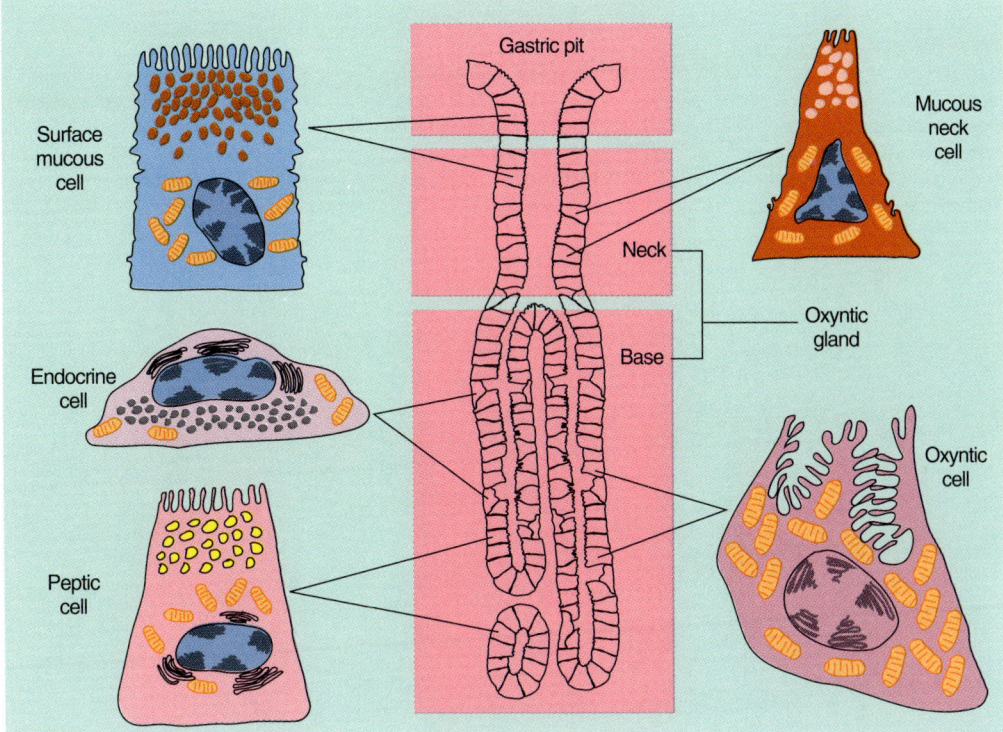

FIGURE 2–2. The oxyntic gland consists of several cell types. The mucous cells secrete mucus and HCO_3^-. The oxyntic cells secrete hydrochloric acid (HCl) and intrinsic factor (IF), and the peptic cells secrete pepsinogen. HCl, pepsinogen, and mucus are propelled along the glandular tube into the gastric lumen to constitute the major solutes of gastric juice. Endocrine cells release peptides into the interstitium that either diffuse into the blood to become hormones or act as paracrine substances.

28 ■ CHAPTER TWO • *Gastric Secretion*

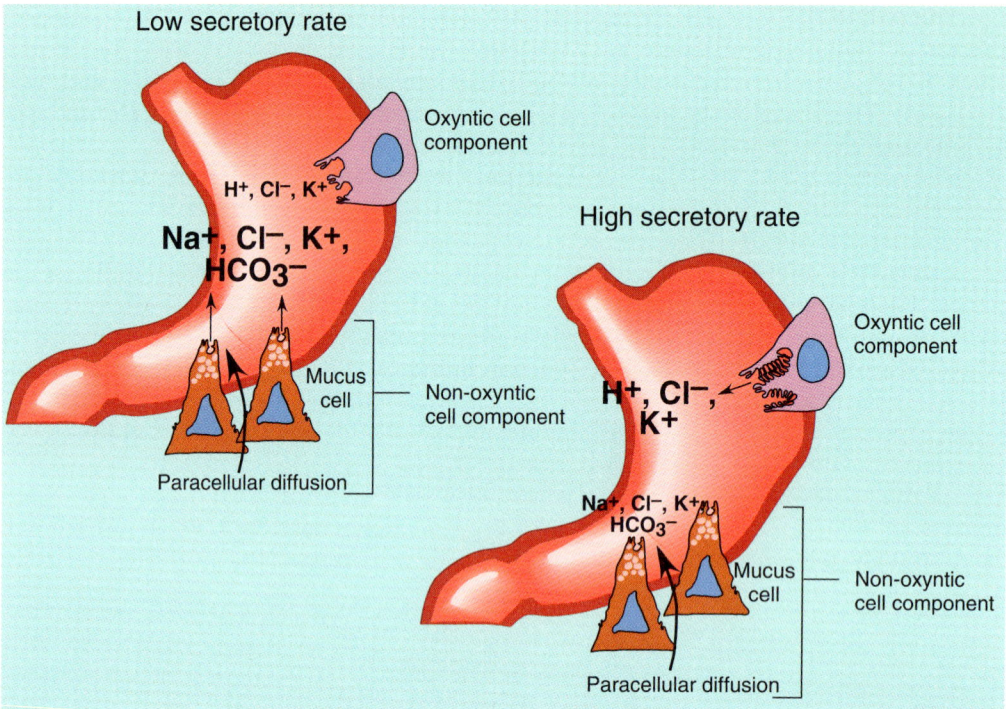

FIGURE 2–3. At any secretory rate, gastric juice is a mix of oxyntic cell and nonoxyntic cell secretions. At low-volume secretory rates, the gastric juice consists mainly of nonoxyntic cell components—namely, mucous cell secretions and paracellular diffusion of interstitial fluid containing mainly water, Na^+, Cl^-, K^+, and HCO_3^- at a pH of 6 to 7. At high secretory rates, gastric juice is derived mostly from oxyntic cells and contains H^+, Cl^-, and K^+ in concentrations quite different from those found in extracellular fluid and has a pH value of approximately 2.

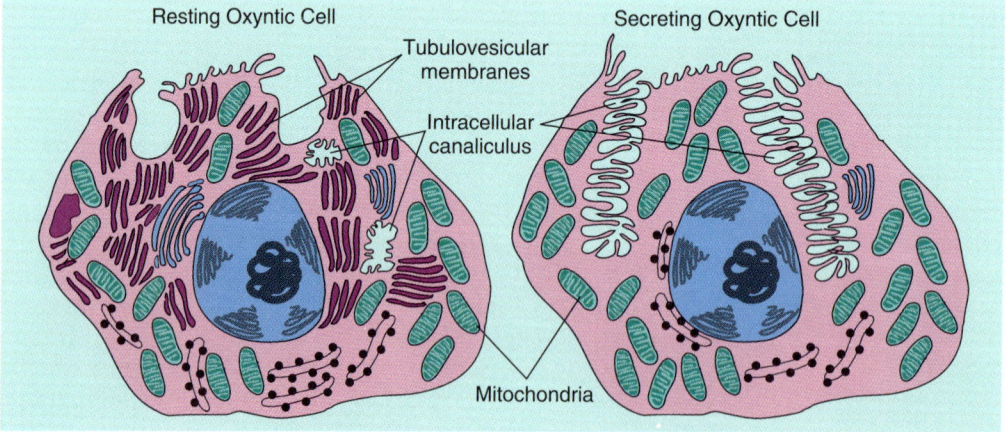

FIGURE 2–4. The appearance of the oxyntic cell changes during secretion. The resting oxyntic cell is characterized by a cytoplasm containing numerous mitochondria, folded membranes, and canaliculi. The secreting oxyntic cell undergoes morphological changes that create an avenue within the cytoplasm for the transport of H^+ across the microvillus membrane and then out of the cell into the glandular lumen.

The cytosol of the resting oxyntic cell contains tubulovesicles, intracellular canaliculi, mitochondria, and many membranes with microvilli (Fig. 2–4). During secretion, the intracellular canaliculi become prominent as a result of a process involving fusion of tubulovesicles and expansion of canaliculi with numerous microvilli. This process increases the surface area available for transport of ions and water. The energy for active transport of protons (H^+) across the microvilli is supplied by the mitochondria.

As stated earlier, oxyntic cells secrete HCl, using an energy-dependent active transport mechanism, and IF, a protein required for the absorption of vitamin B_{12}. Peptic cells secrete pepsinogen, a precursor of the proteolytic enzyme pepsin, which participates in the digestion of dietary protein. Mucous cells secrete HCO_3^- and mucus, which is composed of many different substances such as polypeptides, glycoproteins, and polysaccharides. Mucus and HCO_3^- protect the mucosal lining from damage by acid and pepsin.

Inorganic Secretions

CELLULAR MECHANISMS

The two-component hypothesis explains the variations in electrolyte composition of gastric juice at different secretory rates (see Fig. 2–3). According to this theory, gastric juice is a mixture of a pure oxyntic cell secretion and a nonoxyntic cell component. In the resting stomach, nearly all of the secretion is nonoxyntic in origin. The nonoxyntic component is a mixture of interstitial fluid (paracellular diffusion) and mucous cell secretion. The nonoxyntic cell secretion resembles interstitial fluid in its electrolyte composition: sodium is the major cation, and chloride and bicarbonate are the major anions. On stimulation of the oxyntic cells, the nonoxyntic component is progressively diluted by the much greater volume of acidic juice from oxyntic cells, so that the concentration of sodium decreases to about 5 mEq/L. In addition, the concentration of bicarbonate decreases to zero, because of neutralization by acid from the oxyntic cell with production of CO_2. Pure oxyntic cell secretion consists of H^+ (140 mEq/L), Cl^- (165 mEq/L), and K^+ (20 mEq/L) in an aqueous solution. At peak secretory rates, the gastric juice consists almost entirely of oxyntic cell secretions.

At the basolateral membrane of the oxyntic cell, Na^+ is actively transported out of the cell by the sodium potassium-adenosine triphosphatase (Na^+,K^+-ATPase) (Fig. 2–5). This sodium pump is required because the Na^+ concentration in the extracellular space is three times greater than that inside the cell. Furthermore, Na^+ has to be pumped against the electrical gradient of the basolateral membrane, because the extracellular side is positively charged. At the apical membrane, Na^+ is passively transported into gastric juice, because the intracellular concentration is usually higher than the Na^+ concentration in the juice, and the lumen is negatively charged with respect to the inside of the cell.

K^+ transport is facilitated by its linkage to the active transport of Na^+ and H^+. At the basolateral membrane, two K^+ ions move from the extracellular space into the cell for every three Na^+ ions being pumped out of the cell. The resulting net charge across the basolateral membrane (inside negative charge) attracts potassium into the cell. At the apical membrane, K^+ exchanges for H^+ being pumped out of the cell by H^+,K^+-ATPase. Some K^+ also diffuses passively out of the cell into the lumen in response to both the concentration gradient (i.e., intracellular concentration is about tenfold greater than the concentration of K^+ in the juice) and to the negative charge on the luminal side of the apical membrane.

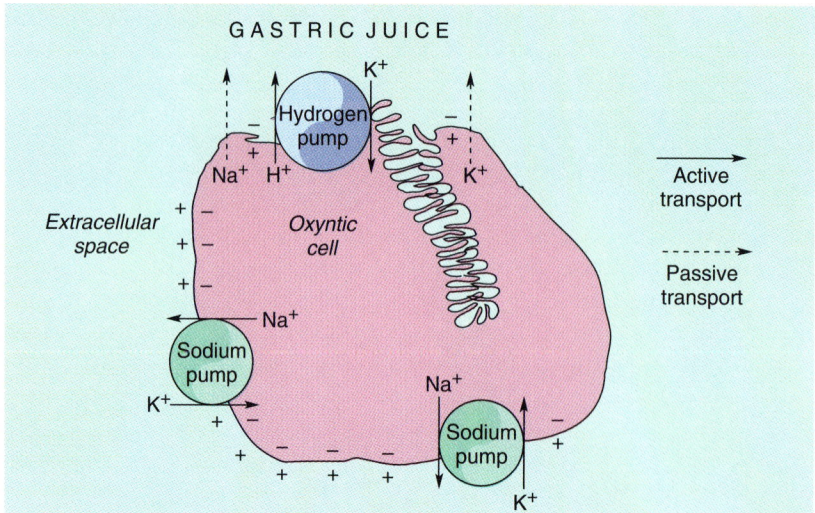

FIGURE 2–5. The secretion of cations into gastric juice involves both active and passive transport mechanisms. The oxyntic cell actively transports H^+ across its apical membrane, exchanging the proton for K^+, which moves into the cell. Both Na^+ and K^+ also diffuse slowly across the apical membrane into gastric juice. At the basolateral membrane, Na^+ is extruded from the cell into the interstitium in unequal exchange for K^+ (ratio, 3 Na^+:2 K^+). The relative impermeability of both membranes to the passive diffusion of K^+ results in the buildup and maintenance of intracellular $[K^+]$ amounting to 160 mEq/L.

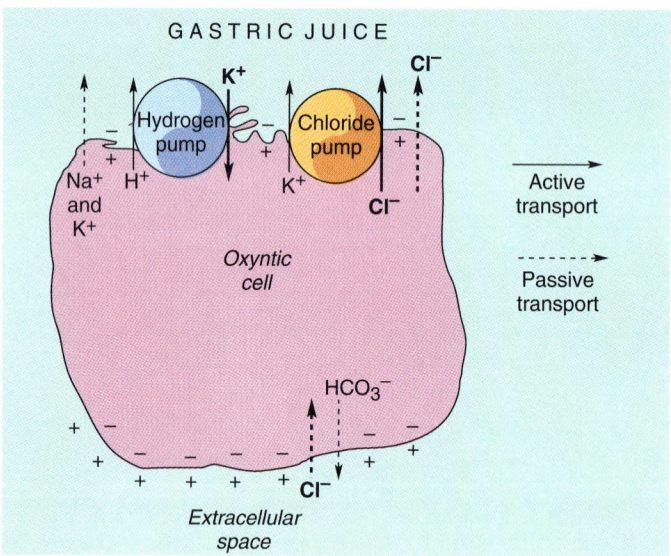

FIGURE 2–6. The secretion of chloride into gastric juice involves both active and passive transport mechanisms. Cl^- is actively transported along with a lesser amount of K^+ into the gastric juice, which causes a negative charge on the luminal side of the apical membrane. Considerable passive diffusion of Cl^- across the apical membrane maintains electroneutrality with the Na^+ and K^+ that diffuse into the juice. Cl^- also diffuses passively into the cell across the basolateral membrane in exchange for HCO_3^-. Because of the large flux of Cl^- into gastric juice, intracellular $[Cl^-]$ is lower than concentrations of this anion in either gastric juice or extracellular fluid.

The movement of Cl⁻ across the tissue compartments of the gastric mucosa utilizes both energy-consuming (active) transport and passive diffusion (Fig. 2–6). At the basolateral membrane, Cl⁻ is passively transported into the cell in response to a concentration gradient (i.e., extracellular Cl⁻ concentration is five times greater than intracellular concentration). HCO_3^- diffuses in the opposite direction. At the apical membrane, Cl⁻ diffuses into the gastric juice to accompany both H⁺, which is actively transported, and the other cations (Na⁺ and K⁺), which are passively transported into the juice. In addition, there is an active transport mechanism for Cl⁻ that pumps the anion into the juice against its electrochemical gradients (i.e., gastric juice Cl⁻ concentration five to eight times greater than the intracellular Cl⁻ concentration, and the luminal side of the apical membrane is negatively charged).

A secretagogue is a stimulant of secretion that binds to a specific receptor on the basolateral membrane of the secretory cell. For oxyntic cells, the three naturally occurring secretagogues are histamine, gastrin, and acetylcholine. Receptor activation by these secretagogues initiates biochemical steps leading to active transport of H⁺ by the oxyntic cell (Figs. 2–7 through 2–9).

Histamine, released into the interstitium by mast cells, binds to the histamine H_2 receptor on the basolateral membrane of the oxyntic cell (see Fig. 2–7). This binding activates an intracellular stimulatory G protein (G_s) that mobilizes guanosine triphosphate (GTP) and adenosine diphosphate (ADP) as energy sources, thereby allowing G_s to stimulate the catalytic subunit of a membrane-bound enzyme, adenylate cyclase. This enzyme converts a small portion of intracellular adenosine triphosphate (ATP) into cyclic adenosine-3′,5′-monophosphate (cAMP). cAMP is responsible for carrying out the secretagogic action of histamine inside the cell and is known as a "second messenger" for histamine. cAMP activates a dependent protein kinase (protein kinase A) that phosphorylates another membrane-bound enzyme, the apical H⁺,K⁺-ATPase. This proton pump hydrolyzes ATP for energy and extrudes H⁺ from the oxyntic cell in exchange for K⁺. In this manner, histamine initiates a train of intracellular events that stimulate the secretion of acid by the oxyntic cell.

Chemicals that inhibit acid secretion can act in several ways at several locations on or in the oxyntic cell (see Fig. 2–7). First, histamine H_2 receptor antagonist drugs (e.g., cimetidine, ranitidine, famotidine) can bind to the H_2 receptor, thereby displacing histamine from receptor binding sites and preventing stimulation of the oxyntic cell by the secretagogue. Second, several naturally occurring agents (prostaglandins E and I, somatostatin, epinephrine) or synthetic drugs (E-type prostaglandin analogues, opiates) can bind to an inhibitory receptor (R_i) and activate an inhibitory G protein (G_i) that suppresses the activity of the catalytic subunit of adenylate cyclase. Finally, drugs that are substituted benzimidazole derivatives (e.g., omeprazole) can occupy the luminal surface of the H⁺,K⁺-ATPase at the K⁺ locus and inactivate the enzyme.

The histamine H_2 receptor stimulates the membrane-bound enzyme adenylate cyclase, which converts ATP into cAMP. Activation of gastrin and cholinergic receptors prompts acceleration of the entry of Ca^{++} from the extracellular space and causes the release of bound calcium inside the cell. cAMP and calcium mediate the effects of many extracellular stimuli inside the cell and are known as "second messengers."

Secretagogues cause the accumulation of two second messengers within the oxyntic cell (see Figs. 2–8 and 2–9). cAMP activates protein kinase A, which causes the phosphorylation of a protein. Phosphorylation is necessary for a conformational change that activates H⁺,K⁺-ATPase, the apical enzyme responsible for transporting hydrogen ion into the lumen of the oxyntic gland. H⁺,K⁺-ATPase hydrolyzes ATP to generate the energy needed for pumping H⁺ out of the cell.

Gastrin and acetylcholine activate the H⁺,K⁺-ATPase by a different mechanism than that stimulated by histamine. Activation of the gastrin and cholinergic receptors prompts

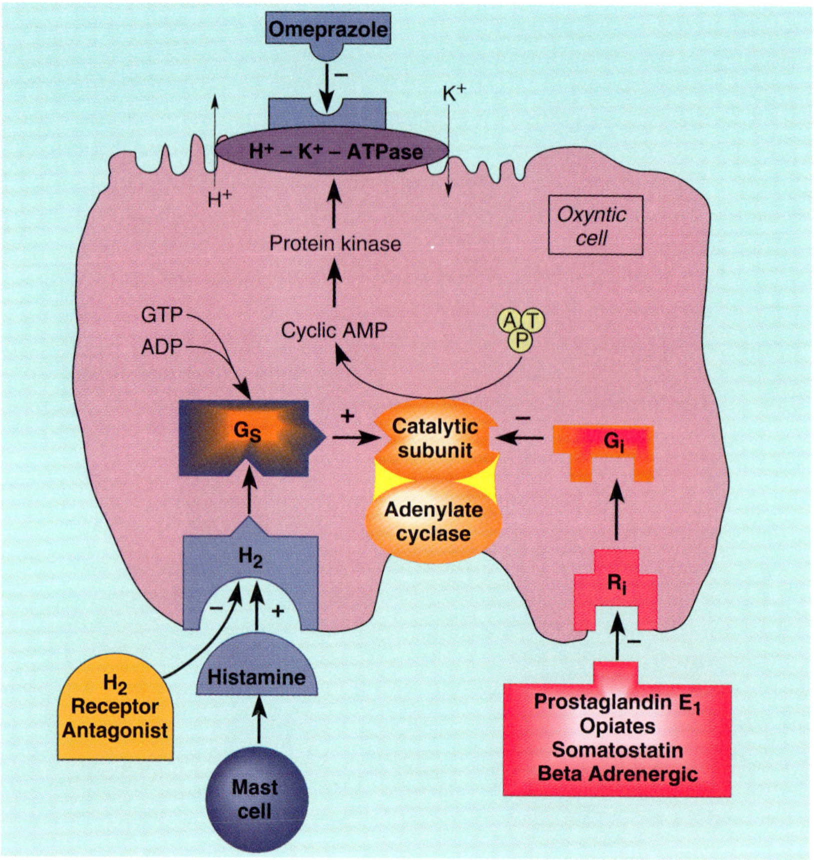

FIGURE 2–7. Adenylate cyclase plays a role in the stimulation and inhibition of acid secretion in the oxyntic cell. The complex cell physiology involved in acid secretion permits several different pharmacological approaches to inhibiting that process. Gastric antisecretory drugs can act in one of three ways: (1) They can occupy the histamine H_2 receptor and prevent its further stimulation, as well as deactivate the stimulatory G protein (G_s) that activates the catalytic subunit of adenylate cyclase; these are known as H_2 receptor antagonists. (2) They can stimulate another basolateral membrane receptor (R_i) that will mobilize an inhibitory G protein (G_i to suppress the catalytic subunit of adenylate cyclase; these include prostaglandin E_1, opiates, somatostatin, and beta-adrenergic agents. (3) They can occupy the K^+ receptor site on H^+,K^+-adenosine triphosphatase (H^+,K^+-ATPase) and prevent its further stimulation; omeprazole is the primary agent.

an increase in available Ca^{++} in the cell. Ca^{++} binds to a protein, calmodulin, forming an active complex that stimulates adenylate cyclase. Ca^{++} also activates protein kinase C, resulting in phosphorylation and activation of the H^+,K^+-ATPase, and additional secretion of H^+ into the gastric juice.

Binding of a secretagogue to its receptor on the basolateral membrane of the oxyntic cell initiates the intracellular events necessary for this cell to secrete acid (Fig. 2–10). These events include increased metabolism of nutrients, beginning with glycolysis and lipolysis, which yields H^+ and energy required for the active H^+ transport into the glandular lumen. Intermediary metabolism of carbohydrate and fat within the oxyntic cell

CHAPTER TWO • *Gastric Secretion*   ■ 33

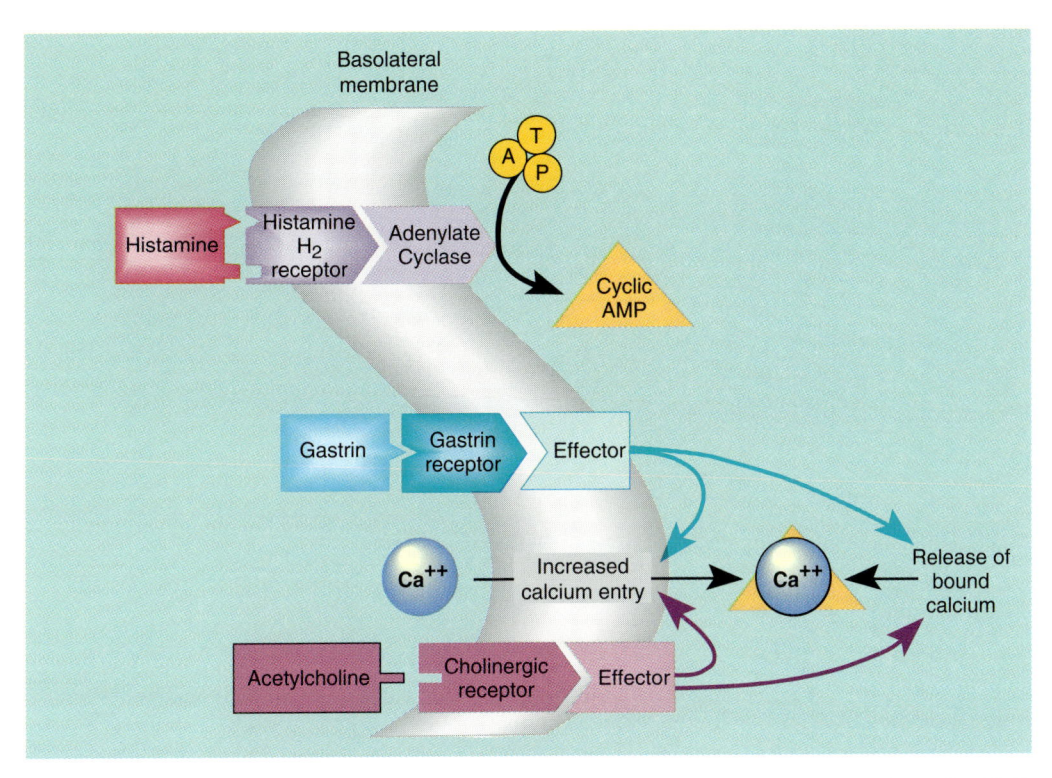

FIGURE 2–8. Secretagogues initiate events within the oxyntic cell that lead to secretion of acid: I. Accumulation of cyclic adenosine monophosphate (cAMP) and calcium. Secretagogues increase the concentration of intracellular second messengers to start processes in the cytosol that lead to H^+ secretion. Histamine stimulates production of AMP; gastrin and acetylcholine stimulate intracellular accumulation of Ca^{++}.

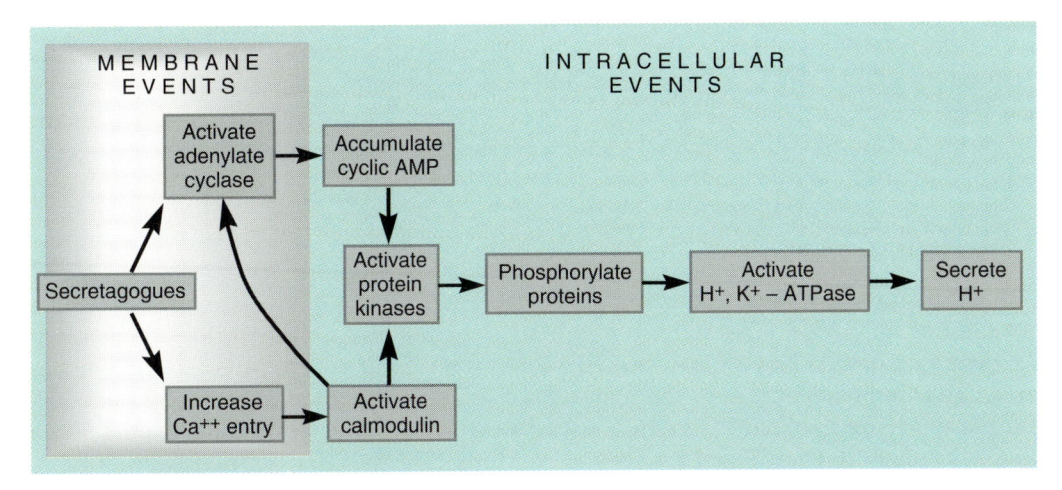

FIGURE 2–9. Secretagogues initiate events within the oxyntic cell that lead to secretion of acid: II. Later reactions. Intracellular Ca^{++} binds to calmodulin and activates protein kinase C. Cyclic AMP activates protein kinase A. These specific protein kinases stimulate phosphorylation of certain proteins, which activates H^+,K^+-ATPase to secrete H^+ into gastric juice.

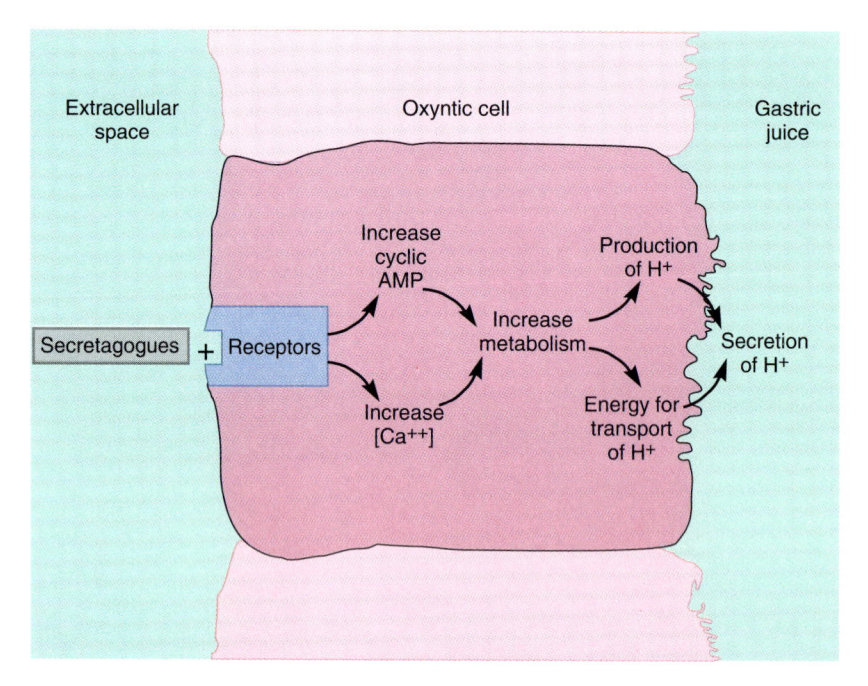

FIGURE 2–10. Secretagogues bind to oxyntic cell receptors and stimulate secretion of acid. The intracellular accumulation of cyclic AMP and Ca^{++} stimulates metabolism in two ways: (1) to produce protons from substrates at the microvilli of the apical membrane, and (2) to generate the adenosine triphosphate (ATP) necessary for transport energy required by ATPase to extrude H^+ into the gastric juice.

produces 4 products: H^+, OH^-, CO_2, and ATP (Fig. 2–11). ATP is hydrolyzed by H^+,K^+-ATPase to provide the energy for active transport of H^+ by the ATPase into the gastric juice. The enzyme carbonic anhydrase converts CO_2 and OH^- into HCO_3^-, which diffuses out of the cell into the extracellular space.

At low secretory rates, gastric juice is predominantly an NaCl solution with low concentrations of K^+ and H^+ (Fig. 2–12). Under these conditions, most of the juice is from the nonoxyntic cell component. As the rate of secretion of gastric juice increases, nearly all of the added juice comes from oxyntic cells, and the ionic concentrations change toward a pure oxyntic cell secretion resembling 0.1 N HCl.

CONTROL

The stomach secretes acid continuously. However, the rate varies greatly depending on the time of day or night and the proximity to eating a meal. When the stomach is at rest, the rate of secretion is quite low. This basal rate is present for most of each 24-hr period and is in great contrast to the high rate of secretion found at mealtime. Basal secretion in the human stomach exhibits a circadian rhythm characterized by a maximal rate in the evening and a minimal rate in the morning. The stomachs of men secrete more acid than the stomachs of women, because there are more oxyntic cells in the male stomach and because female oxyntic cells are less responsive to gastrin.

The three major secretagogues associated with the stomach are acetylcholine (a neurotransmitter), gastrin (a hormone), and histamine (a paracrine substance). When administered exogenously, each secretagogue alone can stimulate the oxyntic cells of the

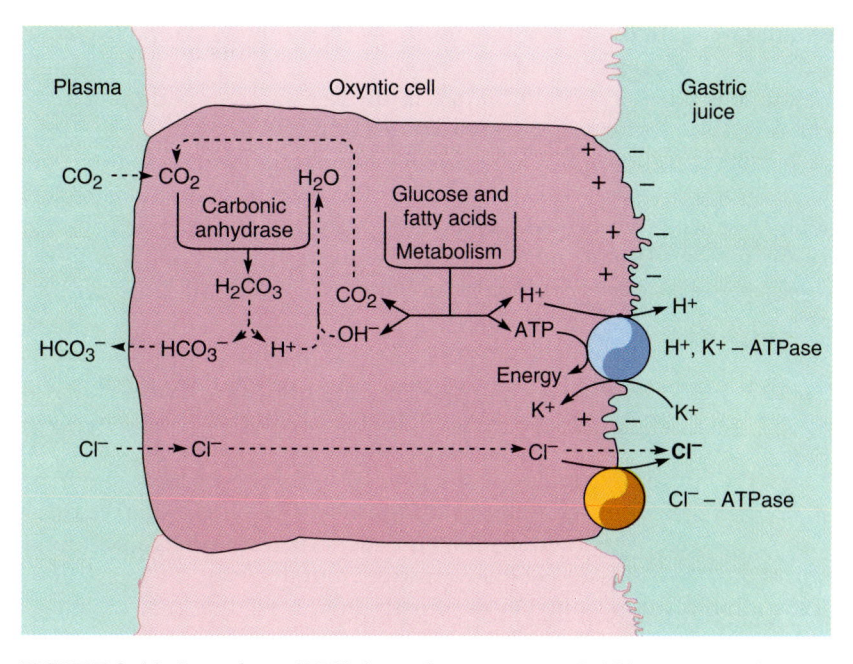

FIGURE 2–11. Secretion of HCl depends on enzymes. Within oxyntic cells, glucose and fatty acids are metabolized oxidatively by enzymes to form H^+, ATP, CO_2, and OH^-. H^+,K^+-ATPase hydrolyses ATP to provide energy for the enzyme to actively transport H^+ from inside the cell ($[H^+] = 10^{-7}$ mol) into the juice ($[H^+] = 10^{-2}$ mol). Carbonic anhydrase facilitates the conversion of CO_2 and OH^- into HCO_3^- and H^+.

FIGURE 2–12. Ionic concentrations in gastric juice vary with secretory rate. At low secretory rates, gastric juice electrolyte concentrations resemble concentrations found in extracellular fluid. As the secretory rate increases, a very unique bodily fluid is produced—namely, acid gastric juice. At peak secretory rates $[H^+]$ = 140 mEq/L, $[Cl^-]$ = 165 mEq/L, $[K^+]$ = 20 mEq/L, $[Na^+]$ = 5 mEq/L, and $[HCO_3^-]$ = 0. The loss of large volumes of acid gastric juice (as in chronic vomiting) without adequate replacement leads to a metabolic alkalosis compounded by hypochloremia, hypokalemia, and dehydration.

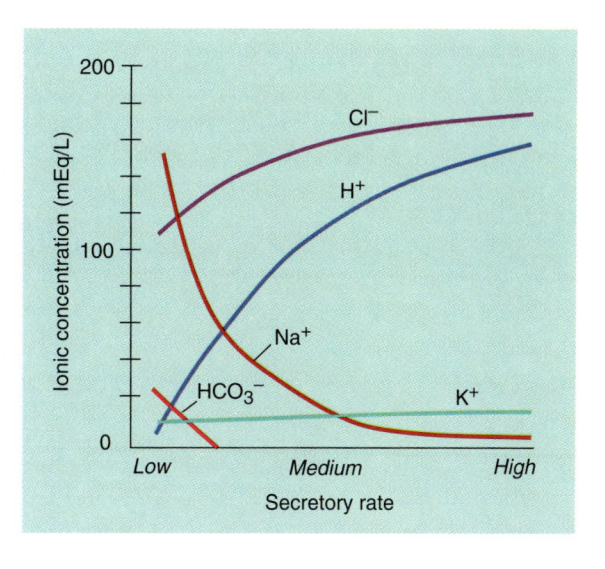

gastric mucosa to secrete HCl. Each secretagogue also occurs naturally in the gastric mucosa. Potentiating interactions between two or three gastric secretagogues serve to amplify the oxyntic cell secretory response. Thus, when histamine binds to H_2 receptors, one result is upregulation of the cholinergic and gastrin receptors, making them more sensitive to subsequent stimulation by their respective secretagogues. Histamine is released from mast cells in the interstitium of the gastric mucosa in close proximity to the oxyntic cell.

The released histamine in the interstitium binds to H_2 receptors on the oxyntic cells. This binding is the initiating step for acid secretion.

Acetylcholine is released from terminals of the vagus nerves and the enteric nervous system located in the plexuses of the stomach wall. Acetylcholine binds to a muscarinic cholinergic receptor on the oxyntic cell, thereby stimulating acid secretion. The G cell in the pyloric gland area releases gastrin into the bloodstream that circulates to the stomach and stimulates acid secretion via a gastrin receptor on the oxyntic cell. All three receptors are on the basolateral membrane of the oxyntic cell. Gastrin is also a trophic (growth) hormone for oxyntic cells and can cause hyperplasia of these cells if it is present in excess, as in Zollinger-Ellison syndrome.

There are three phases of acid secretion during mealtime: cephalic, gastric, and intestinal (Fig. 2–13). Initial stimulation of gastric acid secretion during the cephalic phase is from the sensory response to food (e.g., thinking about, smelling, tasting food). This stimulus triggers impulses in the dorsal motor nuclei that pass to the vagus nerves. Impulses then traverse vagal preganglionic fibers to synapse with postganglionic neurons of the enteric nervous system in the wall of the stomach. The enteric nerves release acetylcholine near oxyntic cells. Vagal stimulation also liberates gastrin-releasing peptide (GRP), which prompts antral G cells to produce gastrin. Neural release of acetylcholine in the antral mucosa inhibits the production of somatostatin, a peptide that inhibits gastrin release. The cephalic phase accounts for one third of total acid secretion by the stomach.

The two primary stimuli for acid secretion during the gastric phase are distention of the stomach by swallowed food and the presence in the gastric lumen of certain chemicals from food, primarily amino acids and peptides. Distention of the stomach produces a vagovagal reflex (i.e., afferent impulses to the medulla and efferent impulses back to the stomach, with both types of impulses carried in the vagal nerve trunks). Distention

Phase of Secretion	Stimulus	Mediation	Secretagogue
Cephalic	Chewing and swallowing food	Vagus nerves; GRP → G cell	Acetylcholine; Gastrin
Gastric	Food distends the stomach	Vagovagal reflex; Local reflex → Acetylcholine	
	Digested protein	G cell	
Intestinal	Digested protein	Intestinal G cell	
All phases		Mast cells	Histamine

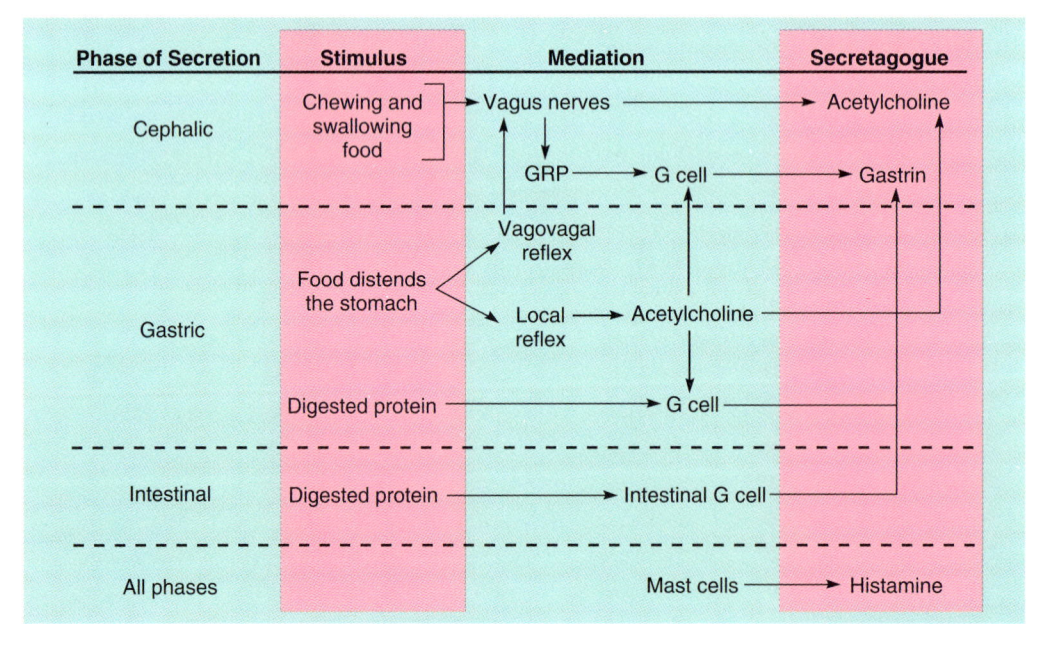

FIGURE 2–13. Three major secretagogues interact during all phases of gastric secretion. During the cephalic phase of secretion, acetylcholine and gastrin are released by neuroendocrine mechanisms. In the gastric phase, other stimuli activate acetylcholine and gastrin release. Histamine is released in all phases of secretion.

also initiates a local reflex via intrinsic nerves in the wall of the stomach. Both distention reflexes are cholinergically mediated. In addition, the local reflex stimulates the G cells of the antral mucosa to produce gastrin. Partially digested protein directly stimulates G-cell production of gastrin and buffers the gastric juice up to pH 3.5, which permits continuous release of gastrin. The gastric phase accounts for half of the total acid secretion.

The intestinal phase of gastric secretion accounts for one sixth of acid secretion after a meal. In this phase, digested protein in the lumen of the gut stimulates upper intestinal mucosal G cells to secrete gastrin into the blood. During all three phases of gastric secretion, histamine released from mast cells also stimulates acid secretion.

Considering that acetylcholine, gastrin, and histamine all induce high rates of secretion, why doesn't the stomach exhibit continuous and excessive secretion of acid? The high rates of acid secretion surrounding mealtimes are reduced to the basal rate of secretion found during interdigestive periods by several mechanisms; these inhibitory processes begin to occur during a meal (Fig. 2–14).

A central antisecretory event is the abatement of hunger with eating, which suppresses the cephalic phase of gastric secretion (Fig. 2–15). During eating and swallowing food, vagal efferent impulses stimulate the liberation of GRP, which releases not only gastrin, but also cholecystokinin (CCK) and glucagon. The last two peptide hormones stimulate vagal afferent fibers, as does swallowed food that stretches the stomach and stimulates local mechanoreceptors. The stimulated vagal afferent fibers release the peptide neurotransmitter substance P in the brain stem. GRP blood levels increase during the meal and stimulate the area postrema of the brain, which relays impulses to the brain stem. This neuroendocrine stimulation of the dorsal vagal complex in the brain stem results in the relay of impulses to the hypothalamic-cortical satiety centers. Their activation prompts a loss of appetite in the eater and eliminates the cephalic phase of gastric secretion. These events, in which eating and swallowing food eventually elicit a loss of appetite, provide a good example of a biological, negative feedback mechanism.

Region	Stimulus	Mediation	Inhibits gastrin release	Directly inhibits acid secretion
Satiety Center – CNS	Eating and swallowing food	Vagal efferents and GRP	+	+
Antrum	Acid (pH < 3.0)	Somatostatin	+	+
Duodenum	Acid (pH < 4.5)	Secretin	+	+
		Nervous reflex		+
Duodenum and Jejunum	Fatty acids	GIP	+	+
		CCK		+

FIGURE 2–14. Several mechanisms terminate the acid secretory response to a meal. The cephalic phase of gastric secretion is terminated by satiety of hunger after prolonged eating and swallowing food. The gastric and intestinal phases of acid secretion are terminated by antral and upper intestinal mucosal responses to secreted acid and to digestion products.

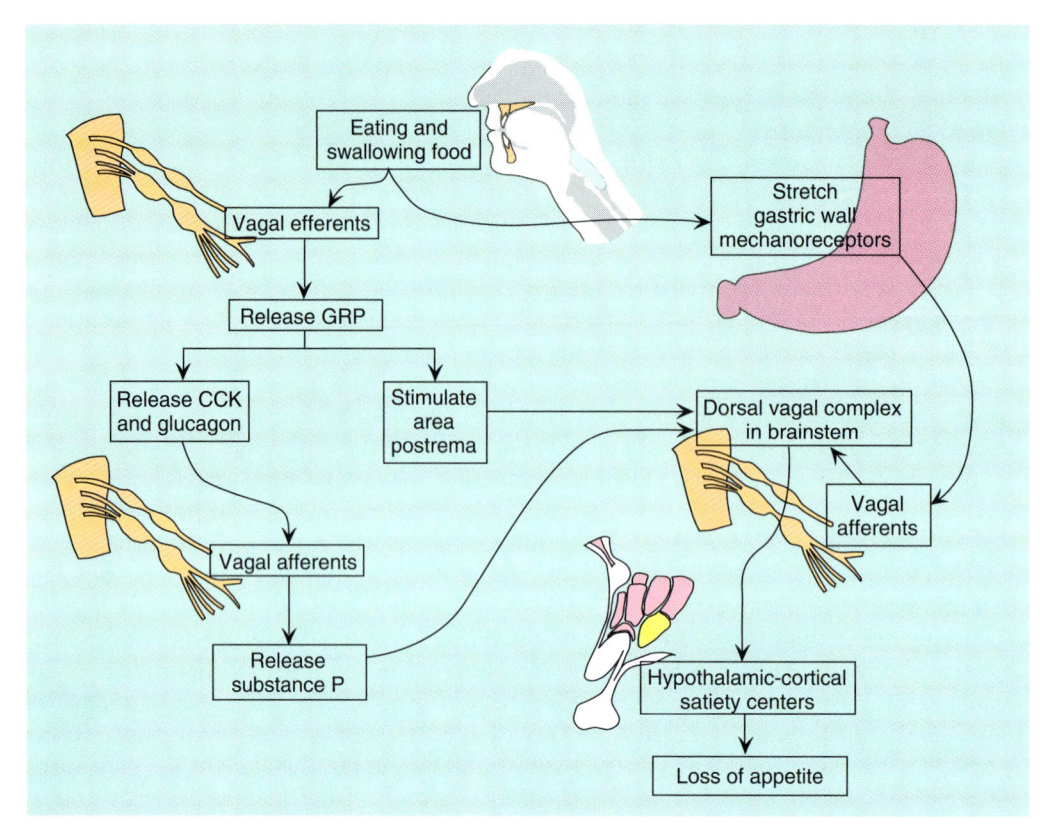

FIGURE 2–15. The cephalic phase of gastric secretion is suppressed by neurohumoral factors. Eating and swallowing food for prolonged periods prompts neural and humoral events that eventually cause loss of appetite, termination of eating, and suppression of the cephalic phase of gastric secretion. The neural components of this negative feedback loop include vagal efferent and afferent nerves, neurotransmitters such as substance P, and higher nervous centers (the area postrema, vagal centers in the brain stem, and satiety centers of the brain). Humoral factors include gastrin-releasing peptide (GRP), glucagon, and cholecystokinin (CCK).

Secretion of HCl by oxyntic cells causes antral mucosal surface pH to fall below 3.0, prompting a second inhibitory mechanism—namely, release of the paracrine substance, somatostatin. Somatostatin decreases gastrin release from the G cells and directly inhibits oxyntic cell secretion of acid (see Fig. 2–14). This inhibitory process is another example of a biological negative feedback mechanism.

Other inhibitory mechanisms come into play when the stomach empties its acid and food content into the duodenum. The emptied stomach cannot use food to buffer antral mucosal pH above 3.0, thereby stopping gastrin release. Acid in the duodenum evokes release of the mucosal hormone secretin, which both inhibits gastrin release and directly inhibits acid secretion. The digestion products of dietary fats in the duodenum cause release of gastric inhibitory peptide (GIP) and CCK, both of which inhibit gastric secretion and contribute to the feeling of satiety. GIP also inhibits the release of gastrin. A neural reflex is induced by acid in the duodenum, which inhibits acid secretion.

Organic Secretions

The three organic components of gastric juice that are of medical importance are mucus, pepsin, and IF.

Mucus is the viscous solution of organic material secreted by mucous cells. The mucus in the stomach and gut is a mixed secretion of different organic substances to which has been added dead, sloughed mucous cells from the mucosal lining. Mucus contains macromolecules such as glycoproteins, other proteins, and polysaccharides. Secreted mucus resides as a thin film (about 50 μm thick) on the mucosal lining and constitutes a protective "unstirred layer." Mucus lubricates the stomach, facilitating the movement of food along the gastric lining and avoiding mucosal abrasions from coarse foods.

The viscous nature of mucus retards the diffusion of pepsin toward the stomach lining, thus protecting the tissue from autodigestion. Glycoproteins in the mucus attract and bind other materials such as water, electrolytes, and lipids. Bicarbonate is trapped by the glycoproteins of mucus and increases the pH in the unstirred layer from approximately 2.0 (in the human gastric lumen) to approximately 7.0 at the mucosal surface. The increase in pH decreases the activity of the proteolytic enzyme pepsin. In addition, the glycoproteins act as decoy substances and are digested by pepsin, thereby sparing the mucosal lining from proteolysis by the enzyme. Mucous cells also secrete lipid into the mucus, which coats the epithelial membranes lining the gastric lumen with a nonwettable surface, thereby protecting the membrane against the action of water-soluble H^+ and pepsin. Vagal stimulation will increase the secretion of mucus, as will coarse pieces of swallowed food that rub against the gastric lining.

Pepsin is secreted as part of a larger molecular weight proenzyme, pepsinogen (molecular weight = 42,500 D). Pepsinogen consists of pepsin and a blocking peptide linked by a peptide bond; it is proteolytically inactive. This peptide bond is pH sensitive, so that at a pH greater than 5.5, the blocking peptide is tightly bound to the pepsin moiety, thus inhibiting its activity. When the pH falls below 5.5, the bond is broken, thereby liberating pepsin. This newly released pepsin then facilitates the cleavage of other peptide bonds to generate still more pepsin, an example of autocatalysis.

The activity of the released pepsin is also pH dependent. In the pH range of 3.5 to 5.5, pepsin displays weak proteolytic activity, disrupting secondary and tertiary structures of proteins. At pH values less than 3.5, pepsin exhibits strong endopeptidase activity, breaking all peptide bonds of ingested proteins except the bond at the C terminal end of the molecule. Ten percent to 20% of swallowed protein is digested in the stomach by pepsin.

Stimulation from the vagal nerves activates the intrinsic cholinergic nerves. This stimulates oxyntic cells to secrete acid into the lumen of the oxyntic gland and peptic cells to secrete pepsinogen (Fig. 2–16). Peptic cell secretion of its proenzyme involves a complex cellular process called "exocytosis," which is discussed in detail in Chapter 3. Acid in the gastric lumen converts pepsinogen to pepsin. H^+ also diffuses back into the mucosal tissues to stimulate the dendrites of the intrinsic nerves, thus establishing a positive feedback loop. Acid in the duodenum causes the mucosa to release secretin, which travels in the blood to the stomach to stimulate pepsinogen biosynthesis and release.

IF is an organic macromolecule located on the tubulovesicular membranes of oxyntic cells (see Fig. 2–4). IF forms a complex with vitamin B_{12} (also called cobalamin) in the lumen of the stomach and duodenum. The B_{12}-IF complex traverses intact through the stomach and the small intestine before binding to a specific receptor on the ileal mucosa; this allows active transport of vitamin B_{12} into the circulation. Vitamin B_{12} is required for hematopoiesis. Failure to absorb adequate amounts of vitamin B_{12} leads to pernicious

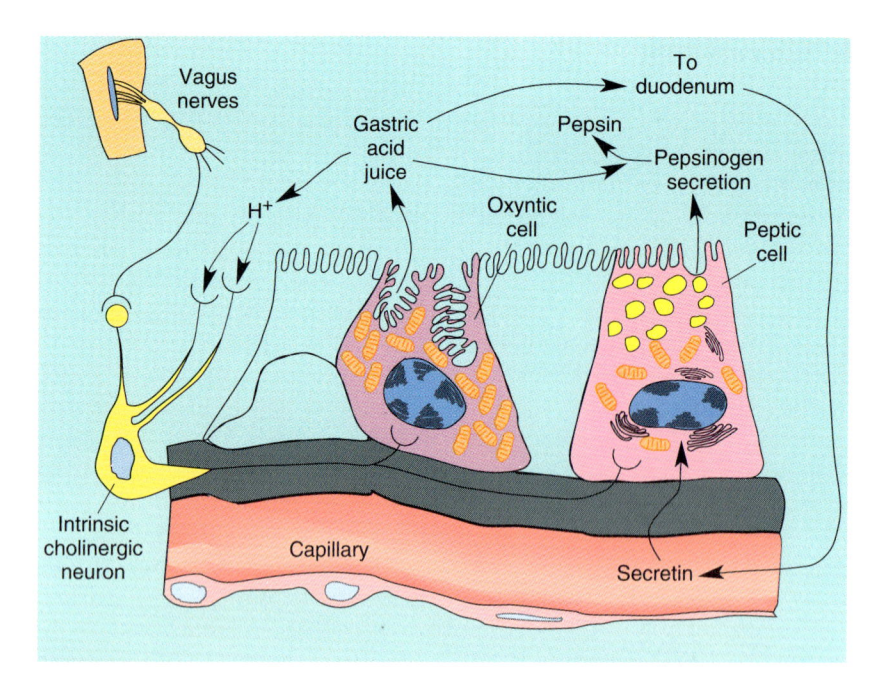

FIGURE 2–16. Secretion of pepsinogen and conversion to pepsin depend on neurohumoral factors and gastric acid. The peptic cell is stimulated by cholinergic neurons in the mucosa. Gastric acid stimulates mucosal cholinergic neurons and evokes intestinal mucosal release of secretin, which also stimulates peptic cell secretion of pepsinogen. Finally, acid converts pepsinogen into the active enzyme pepsin.

anemia, a disease usually caused by deficient secretion of IF coupled with a lack of acid in the stomach.

In patients with pernicious anemia, most often the oxyntic cells, which normally produce both acid and IF, are destroyed by autoimmune processes involving the T-cell lymphocytes, complement system, and circulating antibodies against both IF and H^+,K^+-ATPase. The gastrointestinal handling of vitamin B_{12} is described in more detail in Chapter 7.

Mucosal Injury

Gastric secretion of acid may be abnormally high or low with certain diseases. It is elevated somewhat in duodenal ulcer disease and greatly elevated in Zollinger-Ellison syndrome. Gastric secretion of acid is reduced in pernicious anemia, gastric ulcer disease, and gastric cancer. The most common inflammatory disorders of the stomach are generally termed "peptic diseases." These are disorders involving mucosal surfaces normally bathed by gastric juice (i.e., those surfaces from the lower esophagus to the second portion of the duodenum). The most prevalent peptic diseases are duodenal ulcers and gastritis.

FIGURE 2–17. Breaking the barrier leads to mucosal damage. Normally, secreted H^+ does not move back from the gastric lumen into the mucosa to any great extent because of the relative impermeability of the apical membrane, as well as the neutralizing capacities of the unstirred layer of mucus and bicarbonate and the hydrophobicity of the mucosal surface. Damage to this barrier against H^+ backdiffusion by aspirin, ethanol, or bile allows gastric acid to penetrate the mucosa. The corrosive secretions disrupt mast cells; provoke an inflammatory response; lead to lysosomal proteolysis of mucosal cells; injure capillary endothelium; and prompt ischemia, capillary leakage, and hemorrhage. This type of injury can precede local formation of ulcers. Some naturally occurring substances, such as prostaglandins E and I, protect the integrity of the gastric mucosa against aspirin, ethanol, and bile.

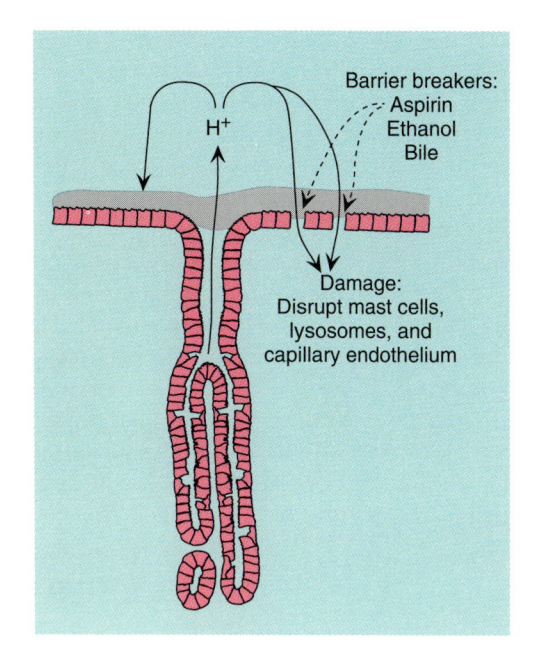

The pathogenesis of duodenal ulcers has been attributed to many causes, including genetic, dietary (i.e., spicy food), and psychological (stress) factors. However, the epidemiological evidence linking these factors to duodenal or gastric ulcers is weak, and the proposed mechanisms are dubious at best. In the case of excessive secretion of acid, it is true that duodenal ulcers in Zollinger-Ellison syndrome are related to the acid overload in the duodenum. However, patients with this syndrome make up less than 1% of the total ulcer population. Patients with duodenal ulcers may secrete more acid than the average for those without duodenal ulcers, but the overlap between the two groups is considerable. Patients with gastric ulcers, by comparison, secrete less acid than the average for the general population, and therefore, it is unlikely that excessive acid secretion is the sole cause of most ulcers. Despite the foregoing considerations, it is also true that inhibition of acid secretion by drugs accelerates the healing rate of both duodenal and gastric ulcers.

Decreased mucosal resistance to acid has also been suggested as another cause of ulcers. The etiology of this decreased resistance is not known and perhaps may be an inhibition of mucus or HCO_3^- formation.

Many substances found in the human stomach have been associated with gastric mucosal damage (gastritis). Bile, if refluxed back into the stomach, acts as a detergent to loosen the membrane bilayer of the mucosal cells. Ingested drugs such as aspirin and indomethacin, provoke punctate bleeding spots in the gastric lining. Ethanol, when applied topically to the gastric lining, damages the mucosa. The bacterium *Helicobacter pylori* has also been associated with duodenal ulcer formation. Nicotine inhibits alkaline pancreatic, duodenal, and biliary secretions, thereby decreasing the pH of the duodenal environment. Prostaglandins and some other substances protect the gastrointestinal mucosae against damage by these agents, a phenomenon called "cytoprotection." Some of the mechanisms underlying the protective effects of prostaglandins against the injurious effects of ethanol and aspirin include stimulation of mucus and HCO_3^- secretion, enhanced mucosal blood flow, activation of epithelial reconstitution over the injured area, and interference with local inflammation by inhibition of neutrophil adherence to endothelial cells.

The aforementioned damaging agents increase the permeability of the epithelial lining of the lumen to the backdiffusion of secreted H^+ (Fig. 2–17). Under normal conditions, the gastric lining is relatively impermeable to protons. When the epithelial lining is injured by topical exposure to injurious chemicals, there is an increase in membrane permeability to H^+, leading to toxic effects on deeper mucosal cells. The damaged mast cells release histamine and leukotrienes, which cause venospasm, hemostasis, edema, and hypoxia. Lysosomes destabilize and release proteolytic enzymes, which act on capillaries, resulting in bleeding. These events can be preludes to ulcer formation.

The main objective in treating patients with peptic diseases is to decrease gastric acidity and allow the peptic lesions to heal. Although gastric acid juice can be neutralized for brief periods with antacids, the major approach medically is to decrease oxyntic cell secretion of HCl with the use of histamine H_2 receptor antagonists, prostaglandins, or benzimidazole derivatives (see Fig. 2–7). These agents inhibit oxyntic cell secretion of acid by interfering with secretagogue receptors (cimetidine, ranitidine, famotidine), mobilizing inhibitory G protein suppression of adenylate cyclase (prostaglandin E_1 analogues), or inactivating the H^+,K^+-ATPase (benzimidazole derivatives).

CASE REPORT: CONCLUSION

CLINICAL IMPRESSION. Chronic duodenal ulcer disease with gastric outlet obstruction, secondary volume depletion, and hypokalemic metabolic alkalosis. Less likely diagnoses would be obstruction from a new lesion, such as gastric ulcer or cancer, or gastroparesis secondary to diabetes mellitus, thyroid disease, or the tricyclic antidepressant.

RECOMMENDATIONS. There was no oral intake until ordered. Four to 5 L of normal saline with potassium chloride added were infused intravenously over the next 24 hr; fluid and electrolyte status was then re-evaluated. Nasogastric suction was continued to decompress the stomach. Amitriptiline was discontinued and the blood glucose level maintained at less than 200 mg/dl with insulin if needed. An upper gastrointestinal endoscopy was performed when the volume and electrolyte abnormalities were corrected.

During the next 2 days, with aggressive hydration, the postural changes in vital signs reversed, Hct decreased to 41%, BUN decreased to 13 mg/dl and albumin decreased to 2.1 gm/dl. The upper endoscopy revealed a normal stomach and esophagus, but the instrument could not be passed through the pylorus into the duodenum. A discrete ulcer was not seen. On the basis of the study, a surgical consultation was obtained. The surgeon recommended a vagotomy and an antrectomy after nutritional repletion with parenteral nutrition. The fasting serum gastrin level was normal.

OVERVIEW

Peptic Ulcer Disease

Probably the most specific symptom of duodenal ulcers is nocturnal pain because of the circadian elevation of basal acid secretion at night. Buffering acid relieves pain, and at night, nothing is available to buffer secreted gastric acid. In about three fourths of patients with a duodenal ulcer, the illness becomes chronic and recurrent. Duodenal ulcer healing and prevention of recurrences using long-term therapy with histamine H_2 receptor antagonist drugs or substituted benzimidazole derivatives do not alter the natural history of duodenal ulcer chronicity and recurrence. That natural history becomes evident on discontinuation of the antiulcer drugs. Ulcer recurrence may be caused by gastric infection with *H. pylori*.

An added complication in the case report was obstruction of the pyloric outflow tract by ulcer-induced scarring. This obstruction had to be differentiated from gastroparesis caused by diabetes or a tricyclic drug. Acid-base and electrolyte abnormalities are characteristic of unresolved pyloric obstruction or protracted nasogastric suction and consist of metabolic alkalosis, hypokalemia, hypochloremia, and dehydration (see Fig. 2–13). Parenteral therapy emphasizes K^+, Cl^-, and volume replacement, which, if adequate, will correct the alkalosis via renal adjustments.

The patient's history also contained some factors that predisposed him to ulcer formation. He smoked cigarettes, which inhibit duodenal bicarbonate buffering of gastric acid. His father and brother had suffered from serious peptic ulcer disease. Furthermore, the patient was under considerable emotional stress and had experienced depression.

CHAPTER THREE

Pancreatic Secretion

CASE REPORT: INITIAL INFORMATION

A 23-year-old man was referred for evaluation of inability to gain weight.

The patient had been thin his entire life. At the time of evaluation he was 5 feet 11 inches and weighed 130 lb, despite previous attempts to gain weight. He ate five times a day, with a typical diet being three eggs, bacon, toast, and milk for breakfast; a protein powder health food supplement at midmorning; two to three sandwiches, ice cream, and a soft drink for lunch; a can of enteric supplement (Ensure) at midafternoon; 8 to 10 oz of meat or poultry, potato or pasta, salad, and dessert for dinner. He denied nausea, vomiting, dysphagia, dyspepsia, heartburn, jaundice, hepatitis, abdominal pain, melena, hematochezia, fever, joint pains, skin lesions, palpitations, constipation, or diarrhea. He described the stools as three to four large, yellowish brown bowel movements a day for as long as he could remember. At times he had observed oil droplets on the surface of the water after defecating. He was disturbed by his thinness, had never induced vomiting after binge eating, and denied the use of laxatives or diuretics. He jogged 2 miles three to four times each week.

Within the preceding year his physicians had obtained thyroid function tests, a blood chemistry panel, a complete blood cell count, a human immunodeficiency virus (HIV) assay, and an upper gastrointestinal series with small bowel follow-through. All findings were normal.

He had been relatively healthy except for routine childhood illnesses and two hospitalizations for pneumonia that lasted several weeks. He was a full-time Ph.D. candidate and did not use tobacco, drugs, or alcohol. There was no family history of bowel disorders, pancreatic disease, or inability to gain weight.

Physical examination revealed an asthenic man with a normal affect and secondary sexual characteristics. His pulse was 70 beats/min, and blood pressure was 110/70 mm Hg. A few coarse rales were heard at the left base of the lung. The cardiac examination was normal. The abdomen was soft and not distended, bowel sounds were normal, and there was no localized tenderness or palpable mass. The liver and spleen were not enlarged. The rectum had no masses, and a Hemoccult test was negative.

PHYSIOLOGY

The pancreas is of vital importance both physiologically and medically. Physically, the pancreas has major digestive and endocrine functions, without which humans cannot survive. Pancreatic juice, which is secreted into the lumen of the duodenum, contains enzymes that are responsible for 50% of the digestion of food. Without such digestion, swallowed nutrients cannot be absorbed. Furthermore, the pancreatic hormone insulin regulates the metabolism of glucose, lipids, and other substrates throughout the body and is essential for life.

The medical importance of the pancreas concerns three prevalent life-threatening or debilitating diseases of the organ: pancreatitis, diabetes mellitus, and pancreatic cancer. Pancreatitis may be acute or chronic, and its pathogenesis is unknown. In this disease, autolysis of pancreatic tissue results in an inflammatory state with local hemorrhage and may result in fatal shock. Diabetes mellitus usually involves either a lack of insulin production because of viral or autoimmune damage to beta cells in the islets of Langerhans (type I) or a genetic defect that produces insensitive insulin receptors throughout the body (type II). Medical problems associated with this disease include accelerated atherosclerosis, coronary occlusion, metabolic acidosis, blindness, stroke, amputation of limbs as a result of poor blood flow, and renal failure. Diabetes mellitus ranks fifth among diseases that cause death in the United States. Cancer of the pancreas ranks fifth among cancer-related causes of death. The cause of this malignancy is uncertain, although some relationship to tobacco and alcohol abuse has been shown. This malignancy is difficult to diagnose early, and when it is diagnosed, it is essentially incurable.

Anatomical Considerations

The pancreas, located deep in the upper abdomen, is embryologically derived from two outgrowths of the primitive gut. Ducts grow into these buds and end blindly in the tissue. The blood supply to the pancreas is derived from pancreaticoduodenal arteries originating from the celiac and superior mesenteric arteries. Separate capillary networks are formed close to the islets of Langerhans and near the acinar cells (Fig. 3–1). The extrinsic neural supply to the pancreas consists mainly of sympathetic and parasympathetic innervation. Postganglionic sympathetic nerves arise from the celiac and superior mesenteric ganglia and follow the arteries supplying the pancreas. These fibers release norepinephrine, a vasoconstrictor substance that reduces blood flow. Preganglionic parasympathetic nerves, which are efferent branches of the vagi, terminate in the pancreas. The postganglionic fibers release acetylcholine, which stimulates secretion of enzymes and production of insulin by the pancreas.

There are three physiologically important cell types in the pancreas:

1. Acinar cells. These are granulated and are located in the pancreatic acini, where they produce digestive enzymes (organic secretion).
2. Duct cells. Theses are not granulated, but are columnar epithelial cells that line the ducts, where they secrete an alkaline solution rich in HCO_3^- (inorganic secretion).
3. Islet of Langerhans cells. These consist of several different types of endocrine cells that synthesize and release peptide hormones into the blood.

Endocrine Secretions of the Pancreas

Pancreatic hormones are produced in the islets of Langerhans, whose most important cell types are the sources of several established and putative peptide hormones and paracrine substances. Alpha cells produce glucagon, a single-chain peptide hormone composed of 29 amino acid residues. Glucagon increases the blood glucose concentration because of two major actions: first, it promotes glycogenolysis, thereby increasing the release of glucose from the liver into the blood; second, it inhibits the activity of pyruvate kinase in the liver, thereby causing gluconeogenesis from alanine.

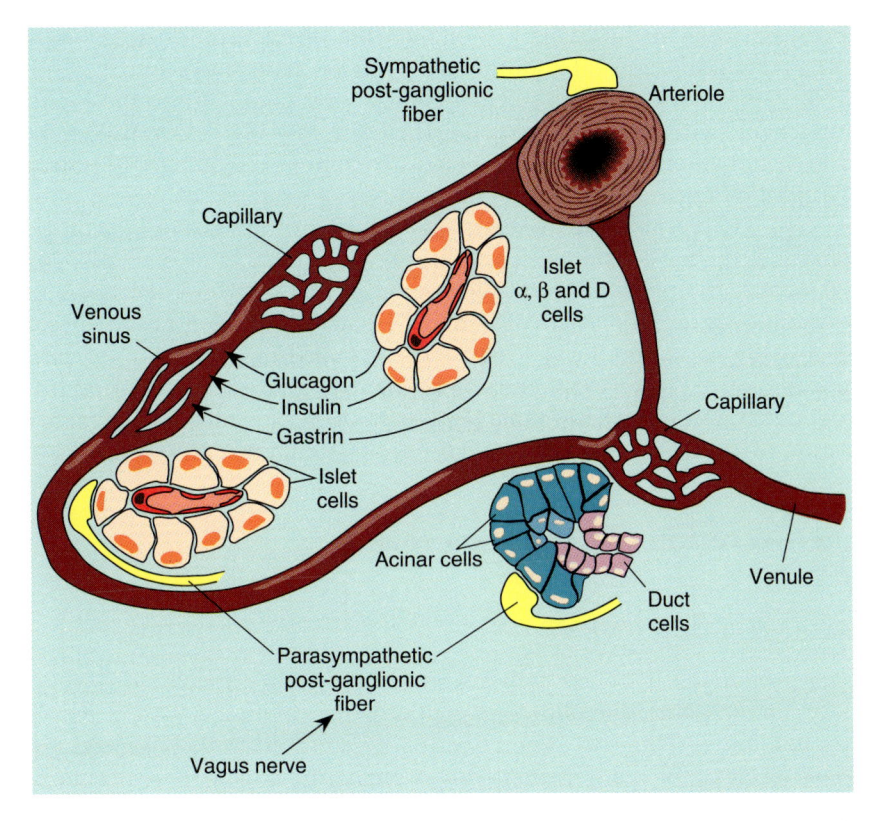

FIGURE 3–1. Histological organization of the pancreas. Separate capillary beds are adjacent to islet cells and to acinar cells and are connected by a portal venous sinus and venule. Sympathetic nerve stimulation reduces blood flow, and parasympathetic nerve stimulation evokes secretion of both islet cells and acinar cells. The islet cells secrete peptide hormones into the venous sinus.

Beta cells produce insulin, which contains 53 amino acid residues. Insulin produces major metabolic effects that lead to a decrease in the plasma concentration of glucose. Specifically, insulin enhances the following:

- Uptake of glucose from plasma into cells;
- Intracellular metabolism of glucose;
- Formation of glycogen in liver, skeletal muscle, and adipose tissue; and
- Inhibition of the conversion of non-nitrogenous, amino acid residues (e.g., alanine) and fatty acids to glucose.

Thus, the actions of insulin and glucagon oppose one another in the metabolism of glucose.

Delta cells produce gastrin, which occurs in several forms, the most common of which in human plasma is a peptide composed of 17 residues. Most gastrin is produced by G cells in the antral mucosa of the stomach. Gastrin is a mild stimulant of acinar cell secretion of digestive enzymes, and it acts as a growth hormone for the gastrointestinal mucosae and the pancreas. Gastrin also stimulates acid secretion from the stomach, contracts the lower esophageal sphincter, and stimulates gastric emptying. The Zollinger-Ellison syndrome occurs when a tumor consisting of delta cells forms or when there is diffuse hyperplasia of delta cells in the islets. In Zollinger-Ellison syndrome, larger than normal amounts of gastrin are produced continuously from the pancreatic source, resulting in a 5- to 10-L/day output of gastric juice. This acidic fluid is emptied into the intestine, producing duodenal ulcers and unremitting diarrhea with loss of K^+. Hypokalemia may lead to cardiac arrhythmias or renal tubular damage. Treatment of Zollinger-Ellison syndrome is aimed at inhibiting gastric acid secretion and involves the use of proton pump blocking drugs (e.g., omeprazole) and even surgical excision of the entire oxyntic gland area of the stomach.

The pancreas also produces two other peptides that appear to be hormones. Pancreatic polypeptide is an inhibitory regulator of exocrine secretion of enzymes by acinar cells. Somatostatin is an inhibitory regulator of endocrine secretion of insulin and glucagon by islet cells. Endocrine tumors of the pancreas have been reported from which excess production of vasoactive intestinal peptide (VIP) occurred, causing severe diarrhea and inhibition of gastric acid secretion; such tumors are known as VIPomas.

Exocrine Secretions of the Pancreas

THE ORGANIC COMPONENT

Enzyme production in acinar cells starts with polysomes attaching to the cisternae of the rough endoplasmic reticulum and synthesizing enzymatic protein on the inside of the cisternal lumen (Fig. 3–2). The enzymes are attached to the cisternal membrane and are inactive. Next, the inactive enzymatic proteins and attached membrane are transported out of the cisternae into small vesicles near the Golgi apparatus. Multiple small vesicles condense into the large vacuole enveloped with Golgi membrane, thereby forming a secretory granule whose contents are inactive at pH 5. When the acinar cell is stimulated at mealtime, the granules migrate to the apical membrane of the acinar cell, where the membrane of the granule fuses with the cell membrane. A hole appears at the fusion site, and the enzymatic proteins are secreted into the lumen of the duct via exocytosis. The enzymes become activated outside the cell in the pancreatic duct, where the pH is 7.5 to 8.0. The foregoing process occurs even in the resting acinar cell, except for the last event—namely, the rupture of the zymogen granules at their point of fusion with the apical membrane. Therefore, in resting cells there is no release of enzymes into the lumen of the duct.

There are two major types of receptors on the basolateral membrane of the acinar cell (Fig. 3–3). The first type includes the cholecystokinin (CCK) receptor and the acetylcholine (cholinergic) receptor. When this type of receptor is stimulated by binding to its respective agonist, there is intracellular conversion of phosphatidylinositol into inositol triphosphate and diacylglycerol. These two intracellular second messengers cause the release of bound calcium from the endoplasmic reticulum, thereby increasing the cytosolic concentration of Ca^{++}. An intracellular protein, calmodulin, binds the Ca^{++}, and the Ca^{++}-calmodulin complex activates the calcium-dependent protein kinase C, which phosphorylates a key protein involved in exocytosis of the acinar cell.

The second receptor type on the acinar cell basolateral membrane binds secretin and causes a stimulatory G protein to activate the catalytic site of a plasma membrane–bound enzyme, adenylate cyclase. This enzyme converts a small amount of adenosine triphosphate (ATP) into another intracellular second messenger, cyclic adenosine monophosphate (cyclic AMP), which then activates the cyclic AMP-dependent protein kinase A. Protein kinase A facilitates the phosphorylation of another protein involved in acinar cell exocytosis.

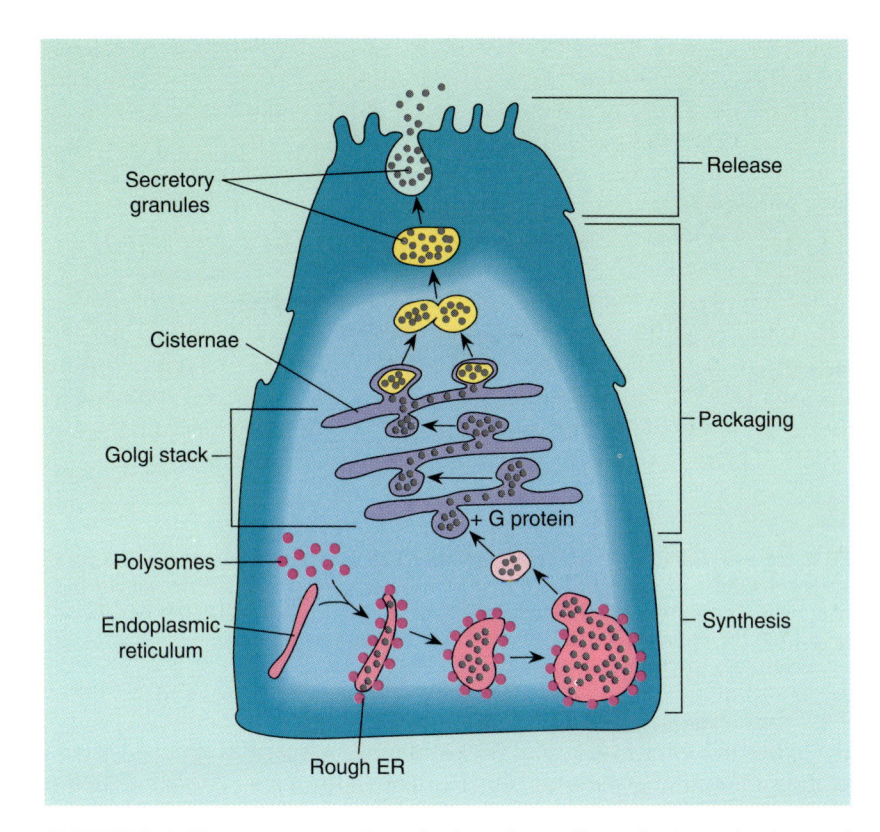

FIGURE 3–2. The secretory pathway in the acinar cell: synthesis, packaging, and release of enzyme. Pancreatic enzymes are synthesized, packaged, stored, and released from acinar cells by the process of exocytosis, which involves multiple subcellular organelles. Most of the packaging of newly synthesized enzymatic protein occurs in the Golgi stack. A G protein facilitates the transfer of enzymatic protein from endoplasmic vesicles into the cisternae. Secretory granules exist in the cytoplasm or migrate to the apical membrane. ER = Endoplasmic reticulum.

Because two separate cellular processes are involved in the stimulation of enzymatic secretion by the acinar cell, the secretagogic actions of CCK or acetylcholine are potentiated by secretin (Fig. 3–4). By contrast, the secretagogic actions of CCK and acetylcholine involve the same cellular process and are only additive to one another.

The pancreas produces several important digestive enzymes that are responsible for about half of overall digestion of nutrients in the gastrointestinal tract. Alpha-amylase digests starch, the most prevalent carbohydrate in the human diet. Starch consists of a long main chain of glucose molecules linked to one another by 1,4 glucosidic bonds. In addition, there are side chains of glucose molecules linked by 1,6 glucosidic bonds to the main chain. Alpha-amylase breaks 1,4 glucosidic linkages in starch molecules, but not the 1,6 linkages and not the 1,4 linkages at the ends of the chain,. Maltose (two glucose molecules), alpha-limit dextrins, and maltotriose (three glucose molecules) are the end products of this breakdown. The first critical step in the breakdown of starch is catalysis by alpha-amylase. However, another step in digestion must occur, because these products cannot be absorbed by the gut. More detailed information about the digestion of starch and its breakdown products appears in Chapter 5.

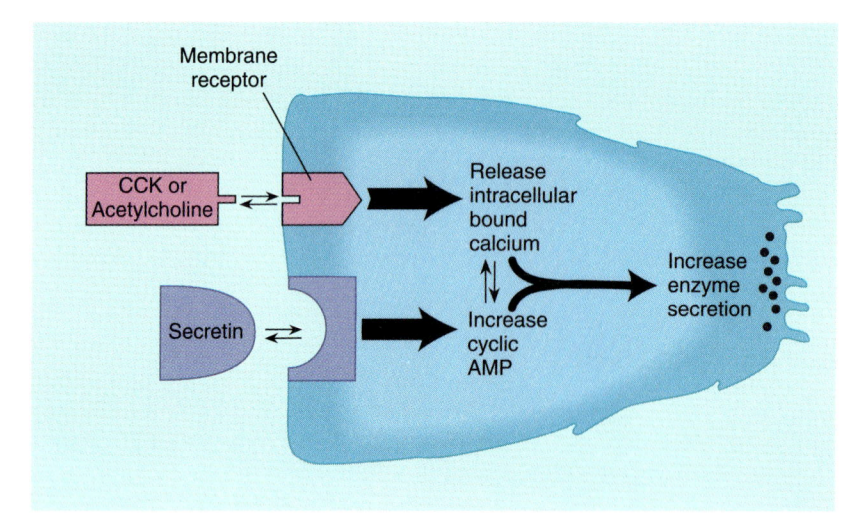

FIGURE 3–3. Stimuli of the acinar cell bind to membrane receptors and initiate intracellular events that increase enzyme secretion. The parallel sets of biochemical events stimulated by cholecystokinin (CCK)/acetylcholine and by secretin are the basis for mutual potentiation of enzyme secretion when all three secretagogues are released at mealtime.

Lipase cleaves the ester linkages of dietary fats. Triglycerides are converted to diglycerides and then to 2-monoglycerides plus two free fatty acids. The latter two end products are absorbed from the intestines. Further information about lipid digestion and absorption is presented in Chapter 6.

Trypsin is produced as trypsinogen, a proenzyme, that is converted to its active form (trypsin) via the action of another enzyme—namely, enterokinase. Newly formed trypsin converts additional trypsinogen molecules to trypsin and is also responsible for conver-

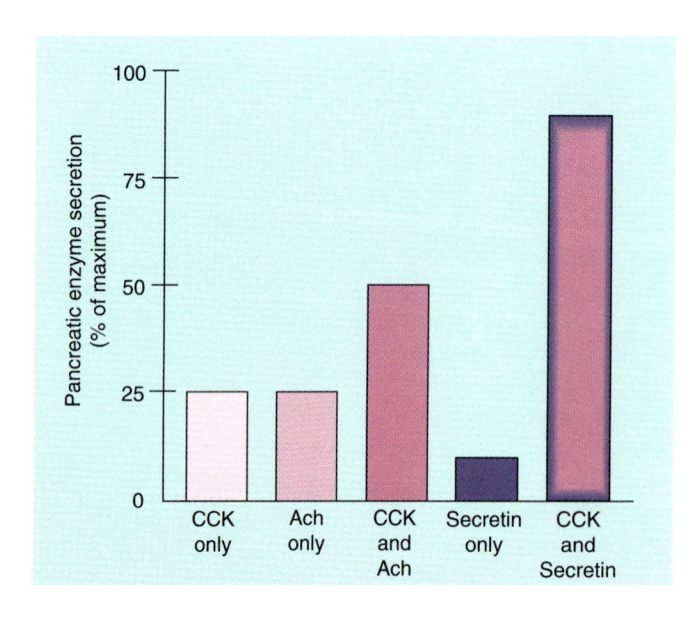

FIGURE 3–4. Secretagogues in combination may produce either additive effects or potentiation. Enzyme secretions stimulated by acetylcholine (ACh) and CCK are additive, whereas secretions elicited by CCK and secretin exhibit potentiation. ACh effects on enzyme secretion are also potentiated by secretin, and the effects of secretin on bicarbonate secretion are potentiated by either CCK or ACh.

sion of other proenzymes to active enzymes. Trypsin breaks down proteins by cleaving primary internal peptide linkages and thus is classified as an endopeptidase. The end products of this process are amino acids, dipeptides, and tripeptides, all of which can be absorbed by the gut. The digestion of proteins and the absorption of protein digestion products are described in Chapter 5.

Carboxypeptidase is also secreted as a proenzyme, procarboxypeptidase, which is converted to active enzyme by trypsin. Carboxypeptidase cleaves C-terminal linkages of proteins into amino acids, which can be absorbed by the gut. Carboxypeptidase is classified as an exopeptidase.

THE INORGANIC COMPONENT

Columnar cells of the duct increase the pH of pancreatic juice up to 7.5 or 8, which facilitates optimal activity of the digestive enzymes. Pancreatic juice also decreases the acidity of gastric contents that have been emptied into the lumen of the duodenum. The duct cell membranes possess three transport mechanisms that affect the electrolyte composition of pancreatic juice (Figs. 3–5 and 3–6). The apical membrane has an electroneutral transporter that exchanges equal quantities of extracellular Cl^- for intracellular HCO_3^-. Thus, stimulation of this apical transporter by increasing the intracellular concentration of HCO_3^- causes a higher HCO_3^- concentration in pancreatic juice.

The basolateral membrane of the duct cell has an electroneutral transporter that exchanges intracellular H^+ for extracellular Na^+; it also has Na^+,K^+–adenosine triphosphatase (Na^+,K^+-ATPase), which actively transports Na^+ out of the duct cell faster than it facilitates the flux of K^+ into the cell where the K^+ is trapped. Therefore, Na^+,K^+-ATPase produces a net potential difference of about 10 mV across the duct cell, with the luminal surface being negatively charged with respect to the basolateral membrane surface. Furthermore, this Na^+ pump keeps the intracellular $[Na^+]$ low, thereby attracting Na^+ from the interstitium into the duct cell via the Na^+/H^+ transporter. The end result is accumulation of H^+ in the extracellular fluid.

Some of the H^+ in extracellular fluid combines with HCO_3^- in the interstitium to form H_2CO_3, which is unstable and dissociates into CO_2 and water (Fig. 3–6). Duct cell

FIGURE 3–5. The resting pancreatic juice consists mainly of sodium chloride and a small volume of water. At rest, the pancreas secretes a small volume of juice whose electrolyte composition resembles that of plasma. The resting pancreatic juice is contributed by acinar cells and by paracellular diffusion.

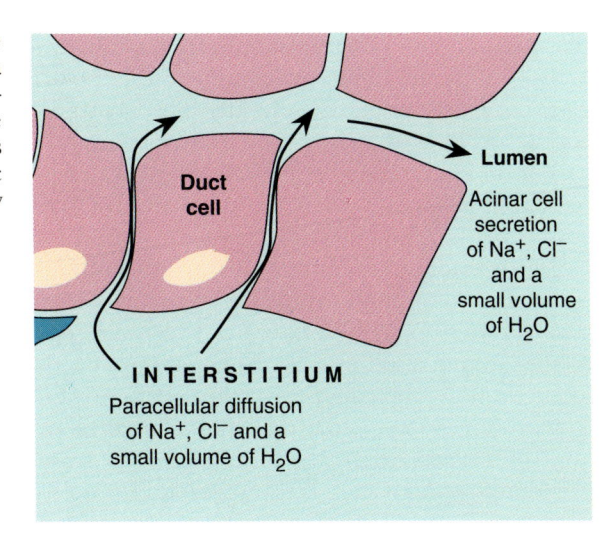

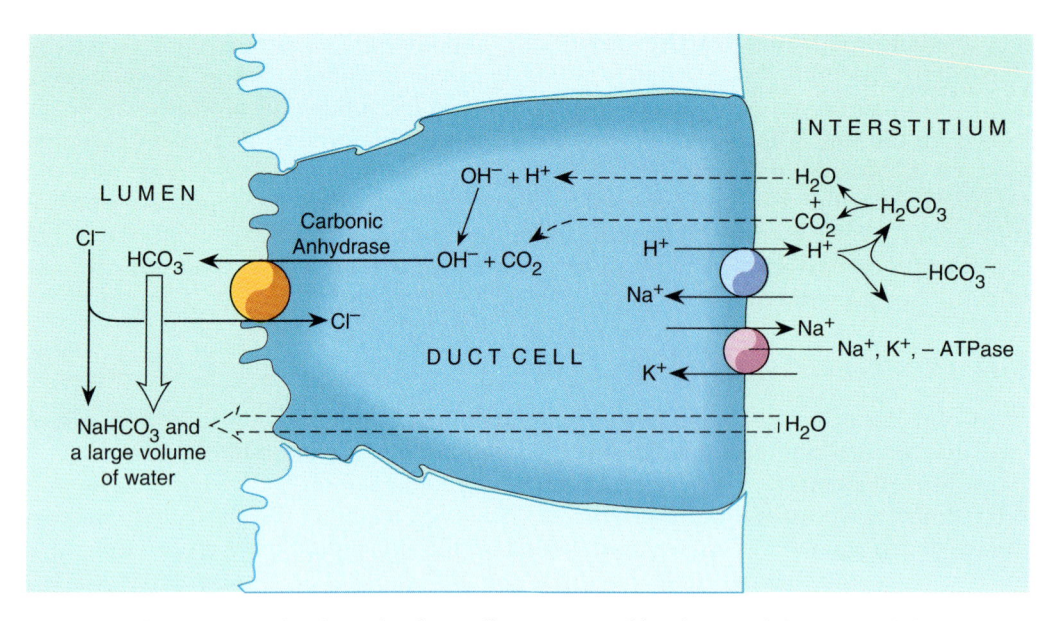

FIGURE 3–6. Mealtime stimulates the duct cell to secrete a bicarbonate-rich pancreatic juice. Stimulated transport mechanisms in duct cells elaborate a large volume of alkaline juice. Carbonic anhydrase in duct cells facilitates the formation of HCO_3^- in the juice.

membranes are very permeable to CO_2, which diffuses readily into the cell and combines with OH^- to form HCO_3^- in a reaction catalyzed by carbonic anhydrase. The intracellular HCO_3^- is extruded into the lumen of the duct in exchange for Cl^-. Na^+, Cl^-, and H_2O can also diffuse into pancreatic juice by paracellular diffusion from the interstitium. As HCO_3^- is moved into the lumen of the duct, H_2O accompanies the electrolyte transport, and the volume of secretion increases.

At low rates of pancreatic exocrine secretion (i.e., between meals), the small volume of acinar cell secretion has an electrolyte composition resembling that of the extracellular fluid (see Fig. 3–5). It is predominantly NaCl, with small amounts of K^+ and HCO_3^-. The quiescent duct cells do little to change that composition. However, in the postprandial period, duct cells are stimulated mainly by secretin, and this stimulation is potentiated by CCK and by acetylcholine. Both CCK and secretin are released by food and gastric juice entering the duodenum. These two hormones and acetylcholine activate Na^+,K^+-ATPase and the other transport events cited earlier, which together lead to secretion of large amounts of HCO_3^- and water into the pancreatic juice. At high rates of secretion, pancreatic juice consists mainly of $NaHCO_3$, with small concentrations of KCl, and its pH is 7.5 to 8.0.

As is evident in Figure 3–7, the concentration of the two cations in pancreatic juice is constant, despite the rate of pancreatic secretion, and is equal to the total concentration of HCO_3^- and Cl^-. However, the concentrations of HCO_3^- and Cl^- are reciprocal relative to one another and are dependent on the pancreatic secretory rate. The venous blood draining the pancreas carries off some of the H^+ extruded from the duct cells and is, therefore, more acidic than the arterial blood that entered the pancreas. This situation is the opposite of that observed in the stomach, where H^+ is secreted into the gastric lumen, and HCO_3^- is transported into the venous blood.

FIGURE 3–7. Bicarbonate and chloride concentrations in pancreatic juice vary reciprocally with secretory rate. As the secretory rate increases, the bicarbonate concentration increases, and [Cl⁻] decreases, despite no change in total ionic concentration. By contrast, [Na⁺] and [K⁺] are stable over the secretory range.

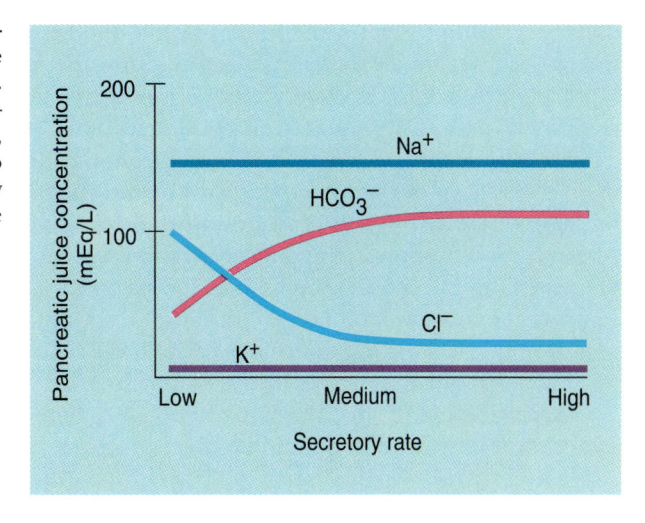

CONTROL

The secretion of pancreatic juice is under combined hormonal and neural control (Fig. 3–8). Secretin is released from mucosal S cells when acid is emptied into the duodenum. This hormone stimulates the duct cells to add HCO_3^- to the pancreatic fluid and potentiates the stimulation of enzyme secretion by CCK (see Fig. 3–4) and acetylcholine. CCK is the most powerful single secretagogue for the pancreatic secretion of enzymes. A duodenal mucosal enterochromaffin cell (I cell) releases CCK in response to digested dietary fat and protein in the lumen of the duodenum and jejunum. CCK also stimulates

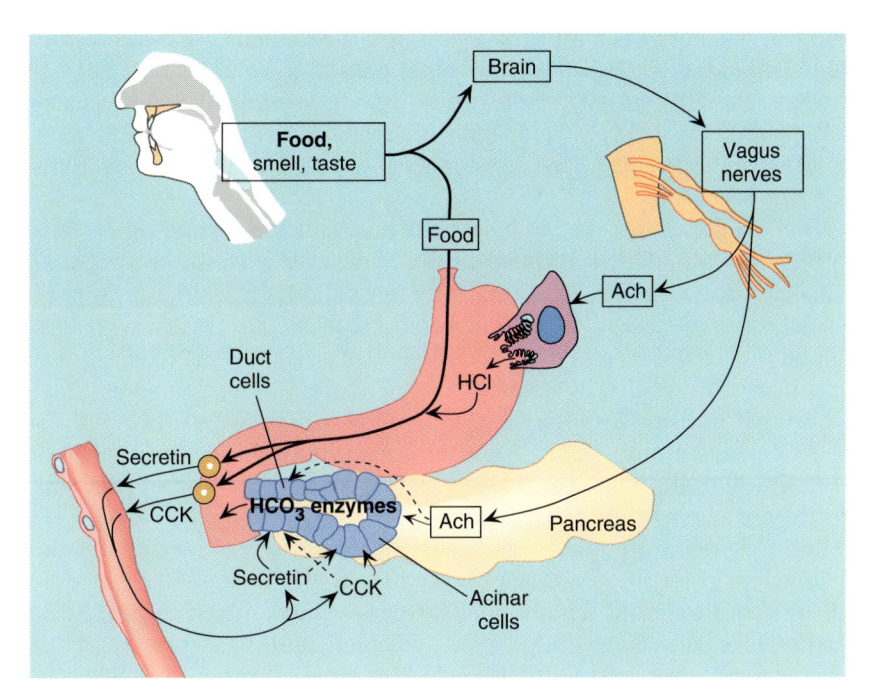

FIGURE 3–8. Control of pancreatic secretion at mealtime involves neuroendocrine factors. The dashed-line arrows for ACh, CCK, and secretin indicate potentiation of stimulatory effects by the other secretagogues on either acinar cells or duct cells.

dietary fat and protein in the lumen of the duodenum and jejunum. CCK also stimulates the gallbladder to contract and eject bile into the duodenum.

Chemically, CCK is closely related to gastrin. The activity of either CCK or gastrin is contained in the C-terminal octapeptide end of CCK and the C-terminal pentapeptide of gastrin. The octapeptides in these two hormones differ by only one amino acid. The remainder of each of the molecules varies from the other considerably, which modifies the biological activity of each hormone in different ways. Thus, CCK produces a far greater stimulus for secretion in the pancreas than does gastrin. Furthermore, addition of gastrin decreases the rate of secretion when the pancreas is being stimulated maximally by CCK (a process known as "competitive inhibition"). Gastrin produces a far greater stimulus for secretion in the stomach than does CCK, and CCK competitively inhibits maximal gastrin stimulation of acid secretion by the stomach.

Acetylcholine, from parasympathetic postganglionic fibers, also stimulates acinar cell secretion of enzymes and potentiates the action of secretin on duct cell secretion of HCO_3^-.

The control of pancreatic exocrine function can also be viewed in terms of phases corresponding to the phases of gastric acid secretion—namely, the interprandial (resting) period and the cephalic, gastric, and intestinal phases of the postprandial period. In the interprandial period, there is a basal rate of pancreatic secretion, which is about 10% of the maximal rate of secretion of enzymes and 5% of the maximal rate of secretion of HCO_3^-.

Acetylcholine is the principal secretagogue during the cephalic phase of pancreatic secretion. Acetylcholine directly stimulates acinar cell secretion of enzymes and potentiates the secretion of HCO_3^- evoked by secretin. The smell and taste of food cause activation of the vagal nerves during the cephalic phase. Bilateral vagotomy reduces the pancreatic response to eating by about half, although the cephalic phase accounts for only one fourth of the total pancreatic secretory response to a meal.

During the gastric phase of pancreatic secretion, distention of the stomach by swallowed food elicits vagovagal reflexes, which stimulate pancreatic secretion via additional release of acetylcholine. This phase constitutes about 10% of the total stimulus for pancreatic exocrine secretion.

The principal postprandial stimulus occurs during the intestinal phase of pancreatic secretion, which accounts for two thirds of the pancreatic secretory response to a meal. The major secretagogues released during the intestinal phase are the most potent stimulants of enzyme secretion (i.e., CCK) and bicarbonate secretion (i.e., secretin). Each of these also potentiates the secretagogic actions of the other. CCK is released by duodenal and jejunal I cells, when the mucosal surface is bathed by certain digestion products namely, the long- and medium-chain (eight or more carbon atoms) fatty acids, the L-isomers of certain amino acids (methionine, phenylalanine, valine), and a few glycine-containing dipeptides. Undigested dietary triglycerides and proteins bathing the I cells do not elicit release of CCK.

Secretin is released from duodenal S cells when the mucosal surface is bathed by gastric hydrochloric acid (HCl) and, to a lesser extent, when the duodenal mucosa is bathed by long-chain fatty acids from digested dietary triglycerides. When the pH at the duodenal mucosal surface falls below 4.5, secretin is released, and the closer the pH gets to 3.0, the greater the amount of secretin that is released. However, only a restricted part of the duodenal mucosa is exposed to a solution at or much below pH 4.5, and hence, very little secretin is released at mealtime. However, even this small amount of the hormone has a potent effect on the secretion of HCO_3^-, because its actions on the duct cells are potentiated by both CCK and acetylcholine. Conversely, secretin potentiates the actions of CCK (see Fig. 3–4) and acetylcholine on acinar cells.

Secretin also protects the duodenal mucosa against the corrosive actions of gastric HCl, because the hormone inhibits oxyntic cell secretion of acid, opposes gastric emptying of acidic juice, and stimulates hepatic and pancreatic secretion into the duodenum (i.e., bile and pancreatic juice contain HCO_3^-). In addition to the antacid effects of secretin, some of the H^+ emptied into the duodenum is absorbed by the mucosa, and some is neutralized by mucosal HCO_3^- secretion into the unstirred layer of the duodenal content. However, the major single factor, that protects the duodenal mucosa against damage by gastric acid is pancreatic secretion of a sizeable volume of juice at mealtime, a juice that contains a bicarbonate concentration four times that of plasma. As a result of these protective mechanisms, the pH at the pyloric sphincter (2.0) increases quickly to 7.0 by the end of the duodenal bulb, a few centimeters distal to the sphincter.

Pancreatic exocrine secretion is reduced to varying degrees by several different human illnesses (e.g., chronic pancreatitis, cystic fibrosis, starvation, kwashiorkor, and an obstructing tumor of the head of the pancreas) and by surgical resection of the organ. When pancreatic secretion of lipase is reduced by more than 90%, dietary lipids will not be digested sufficiently for absorption, and fat will appear in the feces, a condition known as steatorrhea. In steatorrhea from this cause, the fecal fat consists of undigested triglycerides. The stools are larger than usual and are lighter in color, which is characteristic of steatorrheas.

CASE REPORT: CONCLUSION

CLINICAL IMPRESSION. The patient was relatively asymptomatic, and all tests were normal, suggesting that his low weight might be physiological. However, the large bulky stools suggested steatorrhea. The absence of symptoms after eating strongly suggested pancreatic insufficiency rather than small bowel mucosal disease as the potential cause. There was no history to suggest pancreatitis, and if pancreatic insufficiency was documented, adult-onset cystic fibrosis should be considered. Another cause of steatorrhea, hyperphagia due to hyperthyroidism, was excluded by the normal results on thyroid studies, and thus the work-up at this time should be directed toward defining whether fat malabsorption is present.

RECOMMENDATIONS. A 72-hr collection of stool for quantitative measurement of fat excretion on his current diet was undertaken. In addition, a D-xylose absorption test was ordered. Fecal fat excretion was 45 gm/24 hr (normal, 6 gm/24 hr), with a daily stool weight of 1500 gm; D-xylose absorption was normal. The degree of steatorrhea strongly suggested pancreatic insufficiency, and a sweat chloride test was positive. A chest radiograph revealed interstitial lung disease. The patient had cystic fibrosis. Therapy included large doses of high-potency pancreatic enzymes and potential buffering or suppression of secretion of stomach acid.

CLINICAL OVERVIEW

The absence of meal-stimulated steatorrhea or diarrhea in this case suggests pancreatic insufficiency rather than mucosal disease as the basis for the patient's malabsorption syndrome. In pancreatic insufficiency, the key defect in the intestinal handling of food is a lack of digestive enzymes, especially pancreatic lipase. Therefore, most ingested lipids will remain as triglycerides in the gut lumen. In this form, the lipid is not especially irritating to the colonic lining. By contrast, in intestinal mucosal diseases characterized by steatorrhea, the ingested lipid is digested by the pancreatic enzymes into free fatty acids in the gut lumen but is not absorbed. Free fatty acids stimulate colonic secretion of fluid and electrolytes and are metabolized by bacteria to form lactate, thereby lowering intraluminal pH. Hence, after a meal the patient with mucosal disease experiences steatorrhea and diarrhea.

A second pathophysiological consideration stimulated by this case report reflects the great importance of pancreatic exocrine secretion to overall nutrient digestion. Pancreatic enzymes account for about half the digestion of food in the gastrointestinal tract. Hence, profound pancreatic insufficiency is likely to cause serious malabsorption of a range of nutrients that require digestion before intestinal uptake (most proteins and lipids, starch, fat-soluble vitamins, cobalamin, and calcium). However, the pancreatic reserve capacity for enzymatic secretion is great, and frank steatorrhea does not occur until pancreatic secretion is reduced by 90% from normal. Once below this extreme limit of pancreatic insufficiency, severe steatorrhea ensues. Such steatorrhea cannot be totally reversed, even by ingesting maximal doses of pancreatic enzyme preparations extracted from domestic animals.

CHAPTER FOUR

Intestinal Transport of Salt and Water

CASE REPORT: INITIAL INFORMATION

A 37-year-old man came to the emergency room because of diarrhea of 1 day duration.

The patient had been well until 1 day previously, when he developed profuse, watery diarrhea. He had 10 to 15 bowel movements during the previous day and three to four movements the preceding night. There had been no hematochezia or melena. He was mildly nauseated but had not vomited. Abdominal cramps preceded each bowel movement, and there was no fever. He had lost 1 kg weight and was dizzy when changing to an upright position.

The diarrhea had begun the day after returning from a business trip to the gulf coast of Mexico. The patient was a homosexual who had been in a monogamous relationship for 4 years and had tested negative for the human immunodeficiency virus (HIV) 2 years previously. His partner had not been ill. He denied any recent medications or drugs, including antibiotics. He had never experienced such profuse or protracted diarrhea nor had he suffered any other significant past health problems. He did not use tobacco or alcohol. There was no family history of colitis or ileitis.

Physical examination revealed a supine pulse of 100 beats/min, increasing to 120 beats/min on rising; and blood pressure of 130/82 mm Hg that did not change with position. The lips and oropharynx were dry, and the skin over the forehead and triceps tented. The remainder of the examination was normal, including a benign abdomen.

INITIAL LABORATORY FINDINGS. Hct = 42%; WBC = 6900; [Na^+] = 138 mEq/L; [K^+] = 3.1 mEq/L; [Cl^-] = 108 mEq/L; CO_2 = 18 mm Hg; BUN = 30 mg/dl; and creatinine = 1.1 mg/dl. A Hemoccult test was negative.

PHYSIOLOGY

The small intestine is the major site of digestion and absorption of solutes and water in the gastrointestinal system. The gut passively and efficiently absorbs large quantities of water by actively and passively transporting small quantities of solutes, especially Na^+.

The huge surface area of the small intestine is important to its absorptive function (Fig. 4–1). The surface area of the small intestine is increased threefold by the folds of Kerkring, tenfold more because of the villi, and 20-fold more because of the microvilli. The result is 2 million cm^2 of surface area for absorption of fluid and electrolytes.

The surface of the inner lining of the gut is characterized by villi, which are finger-like projections into the lumen of the intestine (Fig. 4–2). At the base of each villus, there

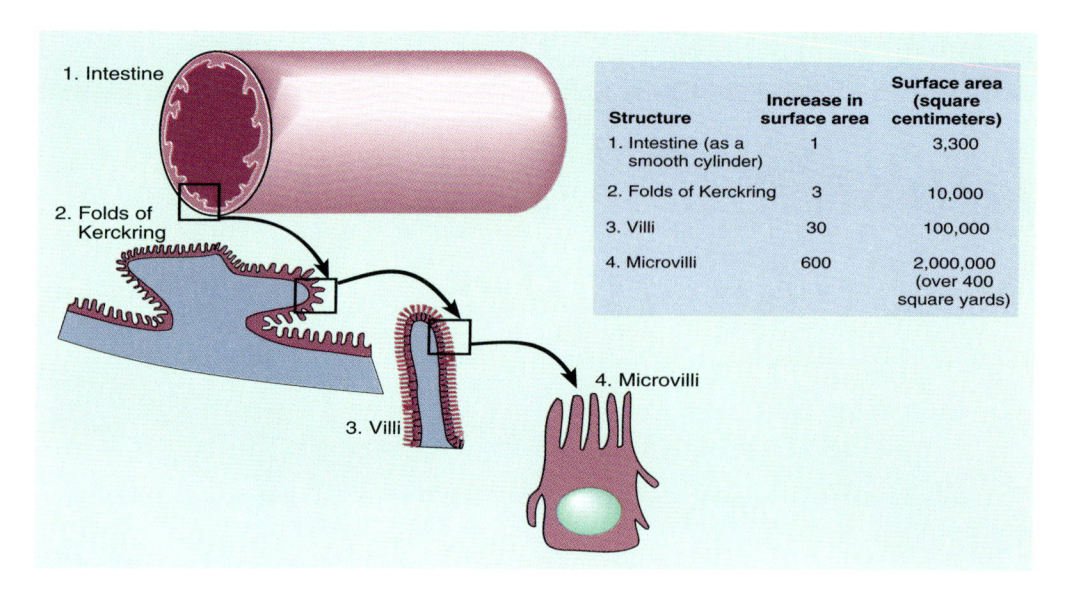

FIGURE 4–1. Intestinal structure amplifies surface area. Transport of solutes and water across a living membrane, such as the small intestinal mucosal surface, depends on the process of diffusion. Diffusion is enhanced by exposing a solution to a larger surface area. In this case, the unique structure of the small intestinal mucosa amplifies the surface area available for absorption of luminal solutes and water by a factor of 600, compared with the flat inner surface of a smooth cylinder of the same length as the gut.

are five to ten crypts. Crypts are tubular pits in the surface of the mucosal lining surrounding the base of the villus. The villus is lined by functionally different cell types, which are continuous with the cells lining the crypts. The villus is about 1.5 mm long, and the crypt is about 0.5 mm deep.

Crypt cells are the proliferative cells of the mucosal lining of the gut, and they also secrete fluid and electrolytes. As these cells migrate along the lining, moving from the crypts onto the surface of the villi, they differentiate into the goblet cells and enterocytes of the villi. Goblet cells secrete mucus and HCO_3^-. Enterocytes mature as they migrate up the villus toward the tip; their microvilli become more pronounced, the activities of their membrane-bound enzymes increase, and their transport processes and carriers develop. These cells also secrete fluids. Enterocytes near the tip of the villus are more active in the digestion and absorption of solutes than are enterocytes near the base of the villus. Functionally, the enterocyte is the most important cell type in the gut with respect to the absorption of nutrients.

As enterocytes and goblet cells migrate up the surface of the villi, they force extrusion of cells at the villus tip into the lumen. This sloughing of older cells constitutes programmed cell death and produces a continual cell turnover. The entire epithelial lining of the small intestine is replaced every 5 days. This rapid turnover of the lining cells is beneficial when an injury to the surface requires repair. However, the rapidly proliferating epithelium of the gut is vulnerable to interventions that are used to attack malignant

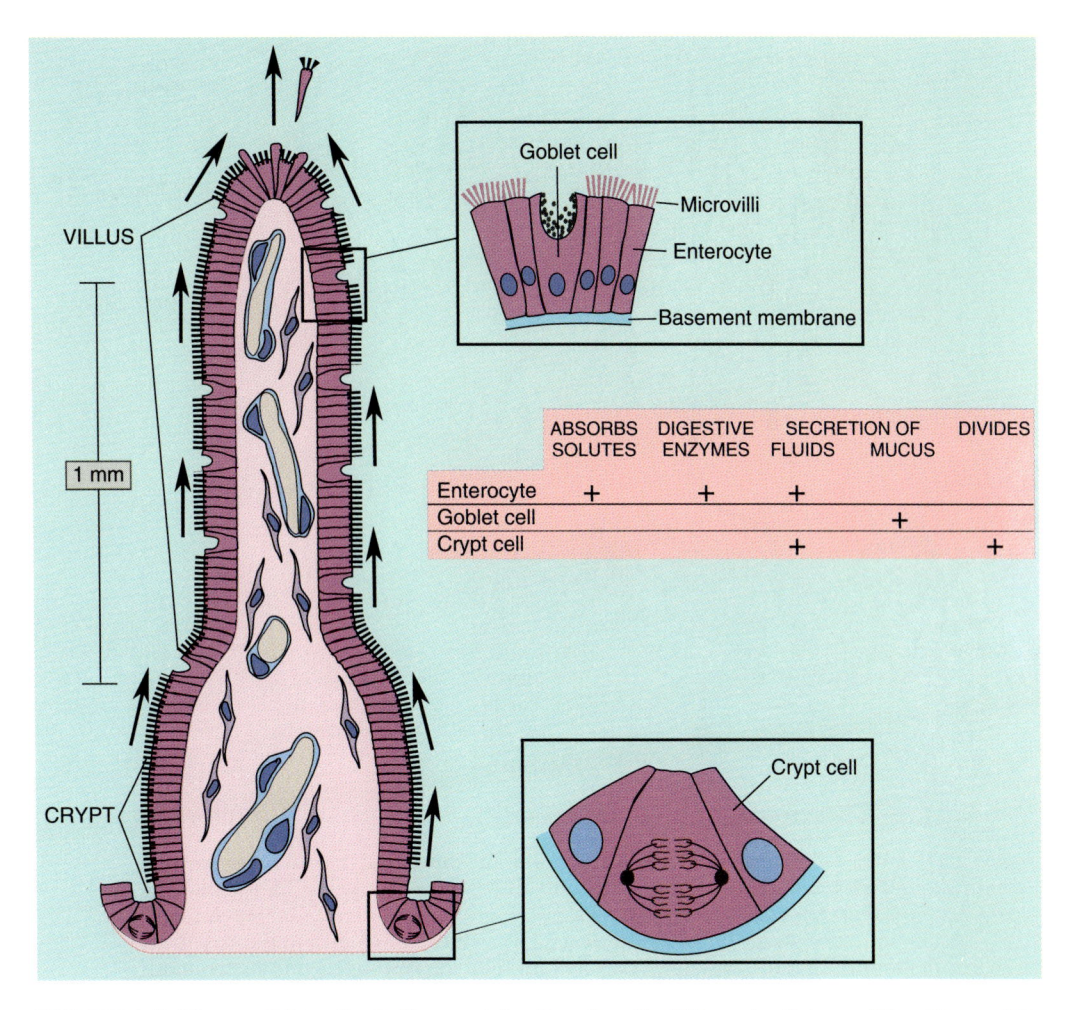

FIGURE 4–2. The small intestinal villus contains functionally different cell types. The villus and its adjacent crypts contain crypt cells, goblet cells, and enterocytes. Crypt cells are germinal and divide to form new cells. Crypt cells and enterocytes secrete fluid into the intestinal lumen, whereas goblet cells secrete mucus. The microvilli of enterocytes contain digestive enzymes and different types of solute transporters.

cells (which also proliferate rapidly). Thus, irradiation or cancer chemotherapy often causes severe damage to the epithelial lining of the gut.

Absorption is the process by which there is a net movement of water, electrolytes, and digested nutrients from the lumen of the small intestine into the mucosal lining. These substances then diffuse into the blood vessels or lymphatics, which carry the absorbed materials to other parts of the body. Secretion is the reverse process (i.e., a net movement of fluid and solutes from the mucosa into the lumen). Substances absorbed from the lumen of the gut must cross several boundaries en route from the lumen to the blood (Fig. 4–3).

The first barrier is an unstirred layer of fluid and solutes that is adherent to the surface of the epithelium. This layer is about 50 μm thick and contains mucus, liquid, and electrolytes, especially bicarbonate. Substances that will be absorbed must diffuse through the unstirred layer before either penetrating the apical membrane of the electrolyte or

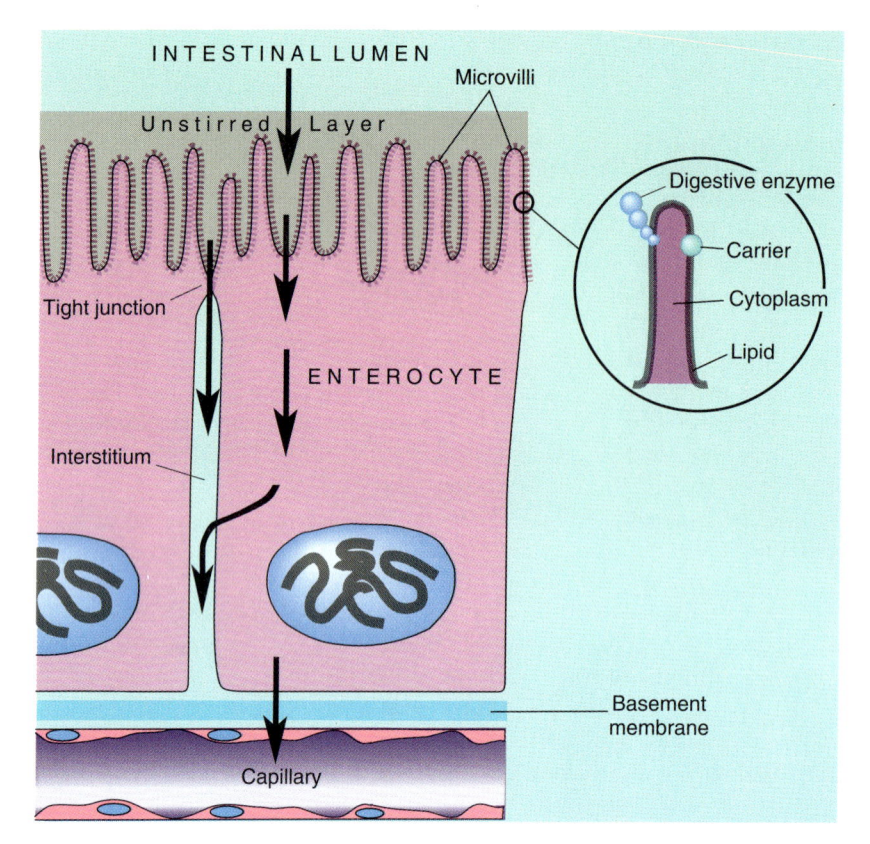

FIGURE 4–3. Substances absorbed from the intestinal lumen cross several boundaries. Solute and water molecules absorbed from the gut lumen into the blood must traverse the unstirred layer, the microvillus membrane or the tight junction, the intracellular matrix or the paracellular interstitium, the basement membrane, and the capillary endothelium. The microvillus membrane contains both digestive enzymes, which extend into the lumen, and carrier molecules, which transport solutes from the lumen into the cytoplasm of the enterocyte.

diffusing through the tight junction between cells. The apical membrane barrier is the glycoprotein–lipid surface coat of the microvilli that contains digestive enzymes and carrier molecules. Carrier molecules transport some electrolytes and nutrients. The next barrier is the cytoplasm of the enterocyte, which contains metabolic enzymes. Then the absorbed substance crosses the basolateral membrane of the enterocyte, which contains transport mechanisms for some ions. Finally, the absorbed material diffuses through the interstitium, crosses the basement membrane, and penetrates the endothelium of the blood vessel or lymphatic.

Types of Intestinal Transport of Solutes and Water

Fluid and electrolytes that diffuse across the tight junctions between enterocytes move directly from the lumen to the interstitial space. This mode of transport, which is called "paracellular diffusion," bypasses the trip through the cell. In the period shortly after eating (i.e., the postprandial period), most fluid is absorbed by paracellular diffusion. Thus, fluid and electrolytes are absorbed by active and passive mechanisms across and around enterocytes (Fig. 4–4).

There are several types of transport across cellular membranes. Passive transport of solutes is caused by electrochemical forces (Fig. 4–5). This type of transport involves no direct expenditure of cellular energy and is caused by diffusion, which is the random movement of particles in a solution. Passive diffusion of water and water-soluble substances across cell membranes involves movement of solute and solvent particles through pores in the membrane. These pores are water-filled channels, about 5 Å (5×10^{-6} µm) in diameter.

Two forces that influence diffusion are the movement of solutes down a concentration gradient and movement of ions down an electrical gradient (see Fig. 4–5). Thus, solutes diffuse from the side of the membrane with the higher concentration of solute to the side with the lower concentration. Cations are attracted to the side of the membrane that is negatively charged, whereas anions are attracted to the positively charged side of the membrane. Lipid-soluble substances can diffuse directly across membranes. The large lipid component of a membrane is permeable to such diffusing lipids, which essentially dissolve in the membrane. Osmosis of water is a special case of diffusion. This passive transport of water through the pores of living membranes is very efficient and is responsible for most water movement across cell membranes in the body. Osmosis allows the transport of huge volumes of water without direct expenditure of energy by the cell on water transport.

Active transport across a membrane requires an expenditure of cellular energy, which drives the movement of solutes against (i.e., in the opposite direction to) a concentration

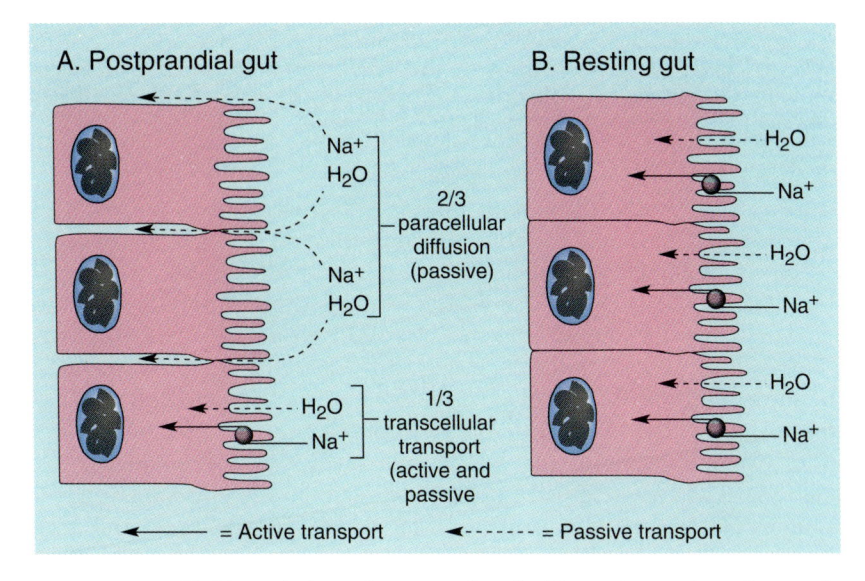

FIGURE 4–4. Fluids and electrolytes are absorbed by active and passive mechanisms across and around enterocytes. *A,* With brisk absorption of fluid and electrolytes at mealtimes, about two thirds of the transport is via paracellular diffusion (i.e., around the enterocytes). The other third of the absorbed material utilizes transcellular transport, which may be active (energy dependent) or passive (diffusion). *B,* During quiescent absorptive periods, the paracellular route of diffusion is not open, and absorption is reduced.

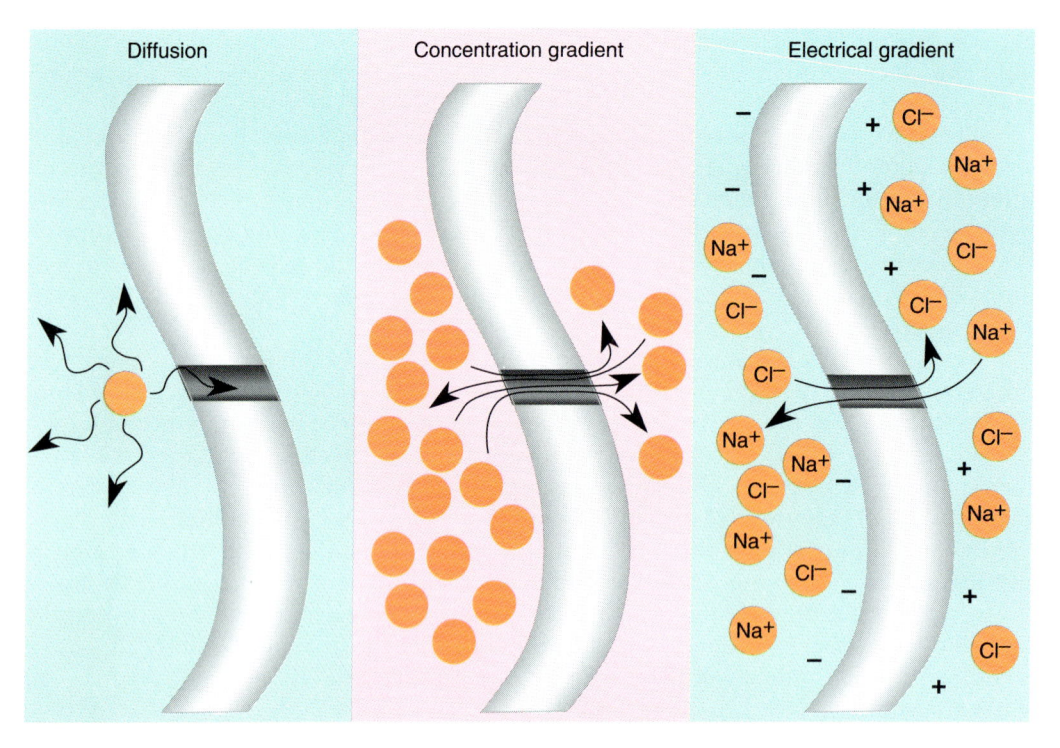

FIGURE 4–5. Passive transport of solutes is caused by electrochemical forces. Diffusion of a solute particle across a membrane involves random movements, with a small probability that the solute will penetrate a water-filled pore of the membrane. Hence, diffusion of solutes across living membranes is slow. A concentration gradient accelerates diffusion in one direction, thereby causing a net movement of solutes. In the middle diagram there are more particles on the left side of the membrane, so there is a net movement of particles from left to right. Another factor that can enhance diffusion of electrolytes from one side of the membrane to the other is an electrical gradient, in which the positively charged side of the membrane attracts anions and repels cations, while the negatively charged side does the reverse.

gradient, an electrical gradient, or both. Active transport involves a special membrane transport macromolecule that is capable of hydrolyzing ATP to get the energy to pump ions against electrochemical gradients. The most common example of such a transport macromolecule is Na^+,K^+-ATPase, also known as the sodium pump. Some nutrient molecules, such as glucose and amino acids, are transported in two steps, the first of which is the binding of the organic molecule, along with Na^+, to a lipoprotein transporter located in the membrane of the microvillus. The second step is a change in the configuration of the transporter that results in movement of the nutrient and Na^+ from the luminal surface of the membrane to the cytoplasmic surface of the membrane, where the cotransported materials are released into the cell. The basolateral membrane of the enterocyte contains Na^+,K^+-ATPase, which actively transports Na^+ from the inside of the cell into the interstitium in exchange for potassium, which enters the cell. Pinocytosis is a special type of active transport for the absorption of large molecules in which the plasma membrane invaginates to enclose the molecules and then pinches off to form an intracellular globule containing the large molecules.

In a usual day, an adult consumes about 1 L of fluid and secretes another 8 L of fluid into the gastrointestinal tract (Fig. 4–6). Of these 9 L which are added to the intestinal

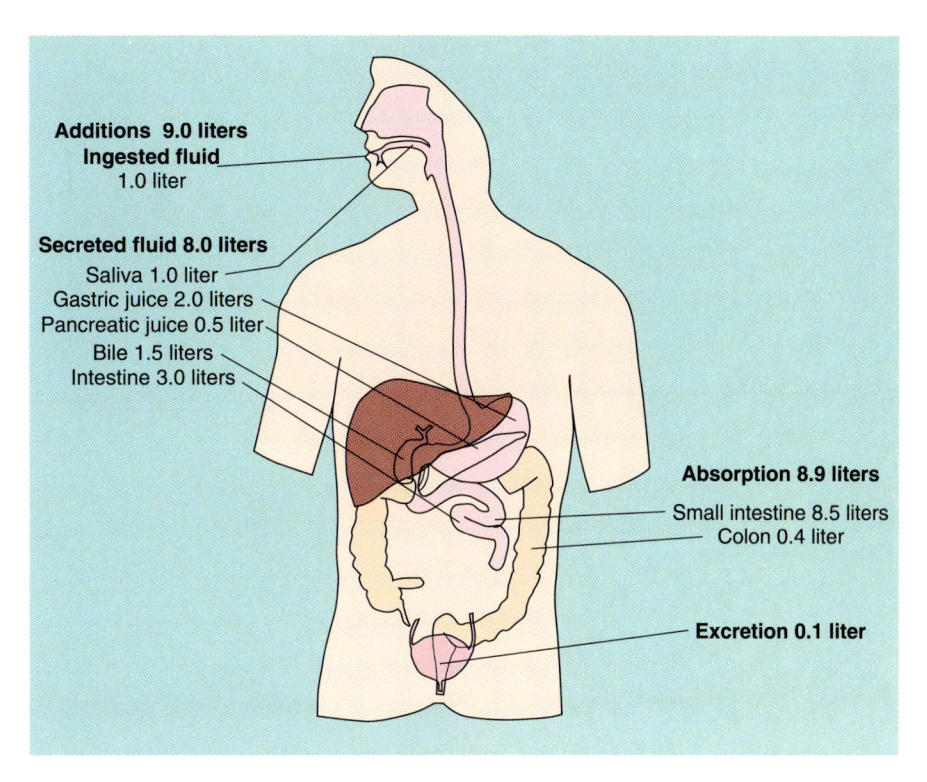

FIGURE 4–6. Ninety-eight percent of fluid added to the gut is absorbed. Every 24 hr an average adult consumes 1 L of fluid and secretes another 8 L into the luminal cavities of the mouth, stomach, and intestine. The small intestine absorbs more than 90% of this fluid, and the colon absorbs about 5%. Less than 2% of the fluid is excreted.

lumen (small intestine and large intestine), 8.9 L are absorbed, mostly in the small intestine. The gut accomplishes this huge absorptive task by taking advantage of the osmotic attraction of solutes such as Na^+ for water.

Upper Small Intestinal Transport of Na^+

APICAL MEMBRANE MECHANISMS

The gut absorbs about 900 mEq of Na^+ daily, with more than 95% being absorbed in the small intestine. Mechanisms involved in transporting Na^+ from the lumen across the apical membrane include the cotransport of Na^+ with certain products of the digestion of nutrients (glucose, galactose, amino acids) by an apical membrane carrier (Fig. 4–7) and a selective Na^+ channel that facilitates Na^+ transport from the lumen. Both the carrier and channel-mediated Na^+ transport are electrogenic (i.e., the transport causes an electrical charge to develop across the apical membrane).

Passive diffusion of Na^+ occurs when the concentration of Na^+ in the lumen is greater than that within the enterocyte. This passive diffusion is a slow process, because the apical membrane is relatively impermeable to the diffusion of Na^+. Na^+ diffusion from the

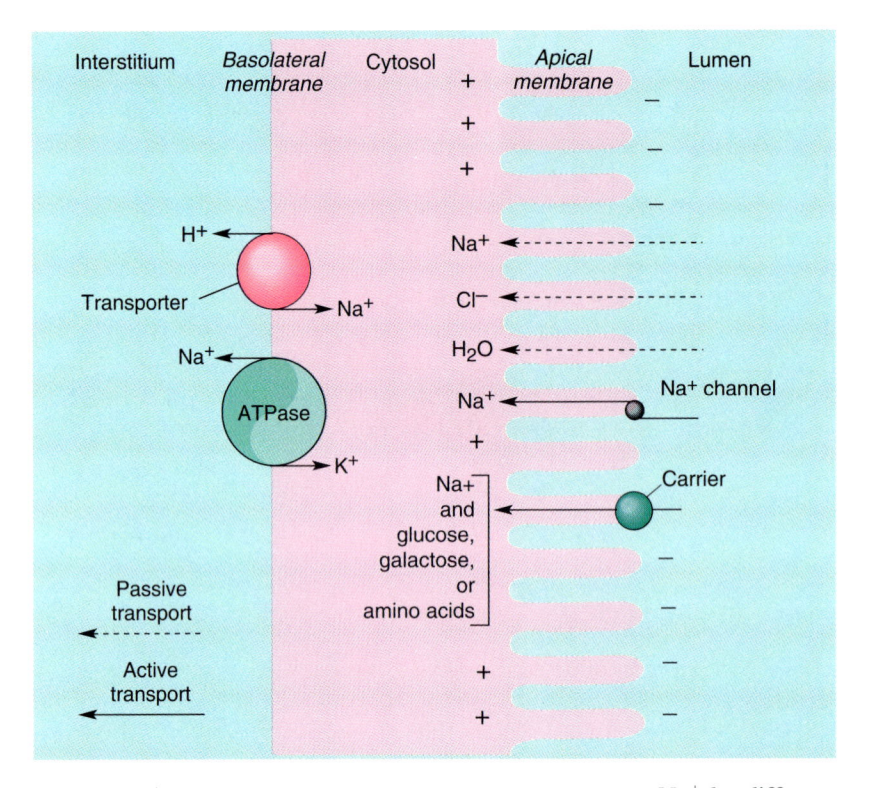

FIGURE 4–7. Upper small intestinal enterocytes transport Na⁺ by different mechanisms. Transcellular transport of Na⁺ across upper intestinal enterocytes involves diffusion, a special Na⁺ channel, and carrier-mediated cotransport of Na⁺ with monosaccharides or amino acids across the apical membrane. Na⁺ movement across the basolateral membrane of the enterocyte involves both the Na⁺,K⁺-ATPase and Na⁺-H⁺ transporter.

lumen into the cytosol is increased by reducing the intracellular Na⁺ concentration; this is accomplished by the basolateral membrane Na⁺,K⁺-ATPase. Nevertheless, this apical membrane impermeability is the rate-limiting step in transcellular movement of Na⁺. Hence, in the postprandial period, most passive diffusion of Na⁺, accompanied by water, occurs via paracellular diffusion. Among the foregoing types of transport, the two mechanisms that are most responsible for increasing Na⁺ absorption (and, therefore, the absorption of H_2O) from the upper small intestine at mealtime are the Na⁺-glucose (or galactose or amino acid) cotransport mechanism and paracellular diffusion. Both processes are enhanced by the digestion of carbohydrates and proteins at mealtime.

BASOLATERAL MEMBRANE MECHANISMS

In the upper small intestine, the basolateral membrane of enterocytes contains two additional mechanisms for Na⁺ transport. A transporter exchanges H⁺ for Na⁺ (i.e., H⁺ is extruded from the cell, and Na⁺ is absorbed into the cytosol from the interstitium). This transporter helps to maintain the intracellular pH at normal levels. The Na⁺,K⁺-ATPase on the basolateral membrane hydrolyzes ATP to obtain the chemical energy needed to pump Na⁺ out of the cytosol and into the interstitium against electrochemical gradients. This energy-dependent, active transport mechanism pumps out Na⁺ in exchange for K⁺, thereby keeping the intracellular concentration of Na⁺ lower than the luminal concentration of Na⁺. The low intracellular Na⁺ concentration attracts Na⁺ from the lumen across the apical membrane via the Na⁺ channel, the Na⁺-glucose transporter, and passive diffusion.

The Na⁺,K⁺-ATPase also pumps Na⁺ across the lateral membranes into the intercellular spaces between enterocytes. When these spaces swell with fluid attracted osmotically by the Na⁺, channels are opened to allow movement of fluid and electrolytes around the cells (i.e., paracellular diffusion) from the lumen into the interstitium. Furthermore, the Na⁺,K⁺-ATPase controls the intracellular fluid volume by regulating the cytosolic Na⁺ concentration. Finally, the absorption of Na⁺ is the driving force behind the absorption of water from the gut. By transporting less than 1 Eq of Na⁺/day from the intestinal lumen into the interstitium, the gut ensures the daily, passive absorption of 9 L of water by osmosis (for each equivalent of Na⁺ absorbed, 55 Eq of water absorbed).

Lower Small Intestinal Transport of Na⁺

APICAL MEMBRANE MECHANISMS

At the apical membrane of ileal enterocytes, there are two exchange mechanisms that are electroneutral (i.e., they cause no net transport of charged ion species in either direction) (Fig. 4–8). One transporter facilitates the movement of Na⁺ into the cell in exchange for the extrusion of H⁺ from the cytosol. A second transporter exchanges the uptake of Cl⁻ for the extrusion of HCO₃⁻. These exchanges are isostoichiometric (i.e., 1 mEq of Na⁺ is exchanged for 1 mEq of H⁺, and 1 mEq of Cl⁻ for 1 mEq of HCO₃⁻). Hence, the elec-

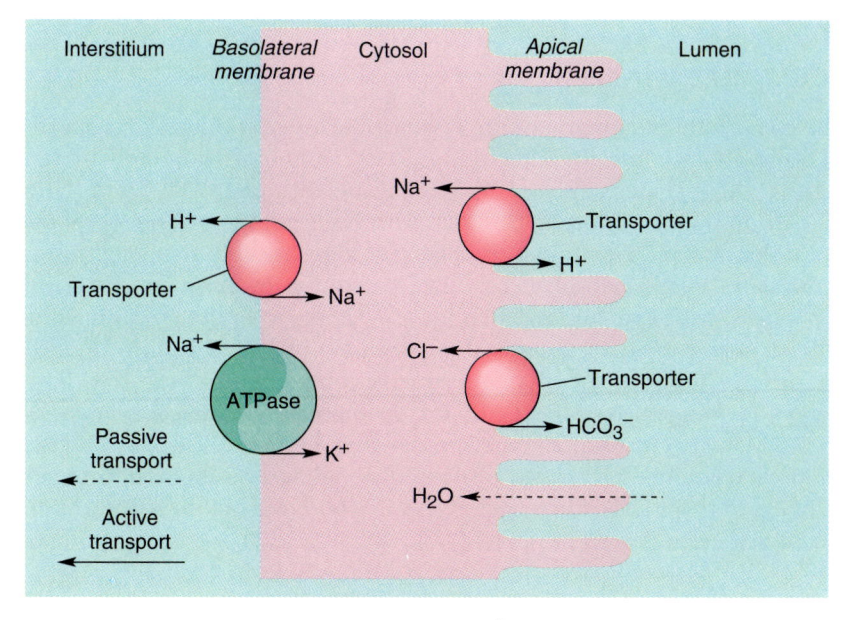

FIGURE 4–8. Ileal enterocytes transport Na⁺ by electroneutral mechanisms. Transcellular transport of Na⁺ across ileal enterocytes involves Na⁺ diffusion and a Na⁺-H⁺ transporter at the apical membrane. This transporter is electroneutral, as is the apical Cl⁻-HCO₃⁻ transporter. The basolateral membrane contains another Na⁺-H⁺ transporter and Na⁺,K⁺-ATPase.

trical currents generated across the apical membrane are equal in both directions. However, the H^+ and HCO_3^- in the lumen react to form H_2CO_3, which dissociates into CO_2 and H_2O. The CO_2 is absorbed into the blood and exhaled in the lungs or propelled down the gut to form part of the flatus, which is expelled to the outside of the body. The H_2O is attracted by osmosis into the enterocyte (transcellular diffusion) or around the enterocyte (paracellular diffusion).

These electroneutral transporters account for ileal absorption of fluid from the lumen, which is important for two reasons. First, these transporters are the main mechanism for the normal absorption of NaCl and H_2O from the gut in the interprandial periods (those periods that are unrelated to eating meals). Second, these ileal transporters are one of two major targets in the gut for certain agents that cause diarrhea in humans (e.g., cholera toxin, *Escherichia coli* toxin, prostaglandins, VIP, and castor oil). When second messengers (cyclic AMP, cyclic guanosine monophosphate [cyclic GMP], Ca^{++}, and Ca^{++}-calmodulin) accumulate excessively in the cytosol of ileal enterocytes, these transporters are inhibited, and absorption of NaCl and H_2O decreases. The other target of agents that cause diarrhea is the crypt cell of the small intestine, which is stimulated to secrete excessive volumes of Cl^- and fluid by the same second messengers.

BASOLATERAL MEMBRANE MECHANISMS

On the basolateral membrane of the ileal enterocyte are the same two transport mechanisms for Na^+ that were described for enterocytes in the upper small intestine; these mechanisms serve the same general functions in both types of enterocytes. The Na^+-H^+ transporter contributes to acid-base balance in the cell by extruding H^+. The Na^+,K^+-ATPase extrudes Na^+ by active transport, thereby keeping intracellular Na^+ concentration low to attract Na^+ from the lumen. The extrusion also expands the lateral intercellular spaces between enterocytes to enhance paracellular diffusion of water and electrolytes.

CRYPT CELL MECHANISMS

On the basolateral membrane of the crypt cell are electroneutral transporters for extruding H^+ and HCO_3^- into the interstitium in exchange for Na^+ and Cl^-, which enter the cytosol. Na^+,K^+-ATPase is also on this membrane and pumps Na^+ out of the cell into the interstitium to prevent cytosolic overload with Na^+ and water. The apical membrane, as well as the basolateral membrane, is relatively impermeable to the diffusion of Cl^-, which accumulates in the cytosol. Accordingly, secretion by crypt cells is normally relatively low because of the rate-limiting step for Cl^- transport at the apical membrane. Any increase in the permeability of the apical membrane to Cl^- will lead to the extrusion of that anion into the lumen of the small intestine, accompanied by both H_2O and Na^+. Cytosolic second messengers (cAMP, cGMP, Ca^{++}) increase the apical membrane permeability to Cl^-. Many agents that cause secretory diarrhea (enterotoxins of *Vibrio cholerae* and *E. coli*, prostaglandins, VIP, castor oil) stimulate an accumulation of intracellular second messengers in crypt cells. Such agents also inhibit electroneutral absorption of NaCl from ileal enterocytes.

Colonic Transport of Na^+

The transport mechanisms of the colonic mucosa are geared to absorb Na^+, Cl^-, and H_2O in exchange for H^+ and HCO_3^- (Fig. 4–9). The last two electrolytes are extruded

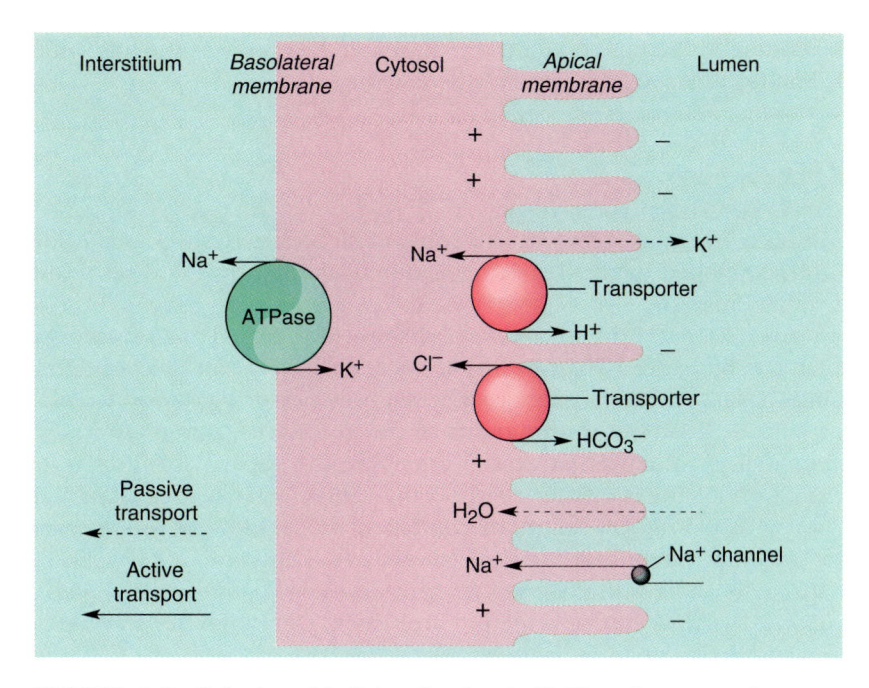

FIGURE 4–9. Colonic epithelial cells absorb NaCl and water and excrete KHCO$_3$. The colonic apical membrane has a Na$^+$-H$^+$ transporter and a Na$^+$ channel to absorb Na$^+$ from the lumen, as well as a Cl$^-$-HCO$_3^-$ transporter to absorb Cl$^-$. Water is absorbed osmotically with these ions. The apical exchange mechanisms transport K$^+$ and HCO$_3^-$ into the lumen, and some K$^+$ diffuses out of the cell in response to both a concentration gradient (intracellular [K$^+$]) and an electrical gradient (negatively charged luminal surface). The basolateral membrane contains Na$^+$,K$^+$-ATPase.

into the lumen, converted into CO$_2$ and H$_2$O, and excreted in the flatus or feces. The apical membranes of colonic epithelial cells contain the electroneutral Na$^+$-H$^+$ and Cl$^-$-HCO$_3^-$ transporters, plus an electrogenic Na$^+$ channel. Hence, there is a net uptake of Na$^+$ from the lumen, and the luminal side of the mucosal lining is negatively charged with respect to the cytosolic side of the apical membrane. This net uptake of Na$^+$ and Cl$^-$ is accompanied by H$_2$O. Excessive concentrations of Na$^+$ in the cytosol are prevented by the Na$^+$,K$^+$-ATPase on the basolateral membrane that exchanges Na$^+$ for K$^+$. The accumulation of intracellular K$^+$ causes diffusion of K$^+$ into the lumen in response to the concentration and electrical gradients.

There is a pH gradient from the cytosol (pH = 5.5) to the lumen of the colon (pH = 7.5). To get rid of excess intracellular H$^+$, colonic epithelial cells utilize the Na$^+$-H$^+$ transporter on the apical membrane. As the intracellular pH decreases, the transporter is stimulated to extrude H$^+$ in exchange for Na$^+$, which is absorbed, along with H$_2$O. There is a linear relationship between Na$^+$ uptake from the lumen by these cells and the size of the pH gradient between the cytosol and the lumen. As Na$^+$ and H$_2$O enter the cell, H$^+$ is secreted into the lumen. This Na$^+$ uptake is saturable (i.e., there is a T$_{max}$), suggesting that the rate-limiting step for the transport is the binding affinity of the transporter for Na$^+$. When the pH gradient between the lumen and the cytosol is reduced, the uptake of Na$^+$ and H$_2$O is also reduced. This reduction in Na$^+$ and H$_2$O absorption will initiate or aggravate a diarrheal state. For example, in isolated lactase deficiency, the undigested lactose is converted into lactic acid by bacteria in the colon; this reduces the pH gradient between the lumen and the cytosol and thus reduces the absorption of Na^+ and H_2O. The result is enhancement of the diarrhea.

DIARRHEA

Diarrhea is a common symptom in people of all ages and has a worldwide distribution. In underdeveloped nations, diarrhea is one of the top three causes of death in infants and young children.

Diarrhea is defined as the excretion of 200 gm or more of H_2O in the stools of an adult during a 24-hr period. The two major types of this disorder are osmotic and secretory diarrheas. Osmotic diarrhea is caused by the presence of excess solute (such as undigested nutrients or laxatives) in the lumen of the gut. Excess solute attracts water from the intestinal wall in volumes that exceed the absorptive capacity of the gut. In osmotic diarrhea, stool osmolality is greater than normal. Secretory diarrhea is caused by crypt cell secretion of isosmotic Cl^- solutions combined with inhibition of electroneutral absorption of isosmotic saline into the ileal enterocytes. This combination exceeds the absorptive capacity of the gut to compensate, and diarrhea results, with the excreted fluid being isosmotic. Diarrhea can be acute or chronic and can range from a mild annoyance to a severe and life-threatening disorder.

Absorption of sodium chloride is inhibited by second-messenger systems in ileal enterocytes (Fig. 4–10). The apical membrane of the ileal enterocyte contains the enzymes (i.e., protein kinases) required to inhibit the absorption of Na^+, Cl^-, and water. The

Disease or stimulus	Membrane mediators	Target enzymes	Second messengers	Inhibitory enzymes
Cholera toxin, VIPoma, PGEoma	Receptor, G protein	Adenylate cyclase	Cyclic AMP	Protein kinase A
E. coli toxin (Turista)	Receptor, G protein	Guanylate cyclase	Cyclic GMP	Protein kinase G
Acetylcholine, Serotonin, Histamine, Neuropeptides, Leukotrienes, Ricinoleate	Receptor, G protein	Phospholipase C conversion of PIP_2 into: 1. Inositol Triphosphate and 2. Diacylglycerol	Ca^{++} – Calmodulin Ca^{++}	Protein kinase II Protein kinase C

FIGURE 4–10. Absorption of NaCl is inhibited by second messenger systems in ileal enterocytes. Pathophysiological stimuli (e.g., bacterial toxins, peptides, prostanoids, amines, castor oil) activate ileal enterocyte surface mediators (e.g., receptors, G proteins), which stimulate membrane-bound enzymes (e.g., adenylate and guanylate cyclase, phospholipase C) to synthesize intracellular second messengers, namely, cyclic AMP and cyclic GMP, Ca^{++}, and Ca^{++}-calmodulin. These second messengers activate specific protein kinases that both inhibit ileal enterocyte absorption of NaCl and stimulate crypt cell secretion of Cl^-. The result is a secretory diarrhea. VIPoma and PGEoma refer to tumors in other organs (e.g., pancreas) that secrete VIP and prostaglandins, respectively, into the blood.

triggering of antiabsorptive enzymes occurs in response to a variety of diseases, drugs, and metabolites, and the symptom produced is diarrhea. The sequence of steps leading to inhibition of absorption in ileal enterocytes is as follows:

STEP 1 The pathological or pharmacological stimulus binds to a receptor on the apical or basolateral membrane and activates a specialized macromolecule in the cytosol that binds high-energy substances needed to activate enzymes. Such macromolecules are termed "G proteins."

STEP 2 The G protein binds GTP as an energy source and activates the catalytic subunit of a critical enzyme such as adenylate cyclase (basolateral membrane), guanylate cyclase (apical membrane), or phospholipase C (basolateral membrane).

STEP 3 Adenylate cyclase converts ATP into cyclic AMP. Guanylate cyclase converts GTP into cyclic GMP. Phospholipase C converts phosphatidylinositol biphosphate (PIP_2) into inositol triphosphate and diacylglycerol. Inositol triphosphate acts on the endoplasmic reticulum in the cytosol of the enterocyte to cause the release of previously bound calcium in the form of ionized Ca^{++}. The conversion of PIP_2 into inositol triphosphate and diacylglyceride also increases the slow inward diffusion of extracellular Ca^{++} through basolateral membrane channels. Some of the intracellular Ca^{++} forms a complex with a calcium-binding protein, calmodulin.

STEP 4 The four cytosolic messengers (cyclic AMP, cyclic GMP, the Ca^{++}-calmodulin complex, and Ca^{++}) accumulate in the apical membrane and activate four membrane-bound enzymes there—namely, protein kinase A, protein kinase G, protein kinase II, and protein kinase C. Diacylglycerol also activates protein kinase C.

STEP 5 The four protein kinases each inhibit electroneutral absorption of Na^+, Cl^-, and water across the apical membrane, leading to diarrhea.

Under normal conditions, as cytosolic $[Ca^{++}]$ increases, absorption of Na^+ across the apical membrane of the enterocyte decreases, and vice versa. Under resting conditions, in the absence of diarrhea, the major rate-limiting regulator of apical membrane absorption of Na^+ is the cytosolic concentration of Ca^{++}-calmodulin, which activates protein kinase II. The latter enzyme phosphorylates the apical membrane–bound protein of the Na^+-H^+ transporter, thereby inactivating this mechanism for absorbing Na^+.

A fluid loss of 10 to 20 L/day can result from cholera. Cholera is the most severe form of diarrheal disease, with an 85% mortality rate during untreated epidemics. However, this mortality rate can be reduced to zero, if patients with cholera are treated adequately and promptly. Cholera is primarily endemic to many tropical areas, is related to contaminated public water supplies and poor hygiene, and is caused by a bacterial enterotoxin from the organism *V. cholerae*. Thyroid and pancreatic tumors may release endogenous VIP and prostaglandins, which produce a less severe form of choleraic diarrhea, acting via a similar mechanism. Cholera enterotoxin, VIP, and prostaglandins stimulate adenylate cyclase to convert ATP into cyclic AMP on the basolateral membrane of the enterocyte. Traveler's diarrhea, or turista, a diarrheal disease common to Western countries, is caused by the enterotoxin of the bacterium *E. coli*, which stimulates guanylate cyclase on the apical membrane to convert GTP into cyclic GMP.

The common mechanisms of secretory diarrhea are the activation of Cl^- secretion (which attracts H_2O and Na^+) by crypt cells and the inhibition of ileal enterocyte absorption of Na^+. Both mechanisms are triggered by the accumulation of intracellular second messengers. The other mechanisms for the absorption of Na$^+$ in the upper small intestine continue to function, but the secretion of Cl$^-$ is much more active, causing a great accumulation of fluid in the gut lumen.

Cholera represents the most extreme example of a secretory diarrhea and rapidly leads to lethal fluid loss and metabolic imbalance. It runs its course in 3 to 5 days, and death is avoided by administering a mixed salt and sugar solution (i.e., a solution containing glucose, NaCl, NaHCO$_3$, and KCl) into the upper small intestine via a nasogastric tube. This therapy utilizes the active cotransport of glucose and sodium and causes the glucose-Na$^+$ solution to be absorbed more rapidly than fluid can be lost by the secretion of Cl$^-$ from the crypt cells (Fig. 4–11).

CASE REPORT: CONCLUSION

CLINICAL IMPRESSION. Acute secretory diarrhea, likely caused by enterotoxigenic *E. coli*, with associated dehydration. The patient was at risk for many other causes of diarrhea—namely, the diarrheogenic organisms found in Mexico or associated with a gay male lifestyle (e.g., *Campylobacter, Aeromonas, Shigella, Salmonella, Entamoeba histolytica, Giardia*), organisms found on the gulf coast (*Vibrio parahaemolyticus*), or unusual organisms more commonly associated with immunosuppression (*Cryptosporidium microsporida*).

RECOMMENDATIONS. Initial diagnostic studies (e.g., stool for routine culture, including *Vibrio*, ova, and parasites) attempted to exclude other, less likely, causes of traveler's diarrhea. In an afebrile patient without blood in the stool, consideration

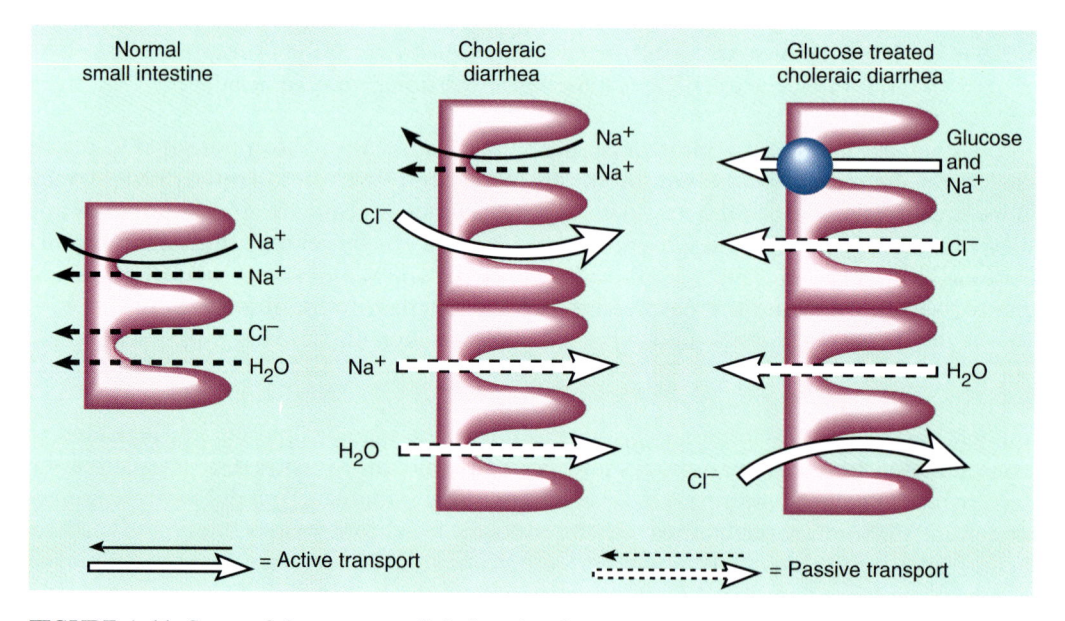

FIGURE 4–11. Successful treatment of cholera involves overcoming secretion of Cl$^-$ with absorption of Na$^+$ and glucose. Normally, the small intestine utilizes active transport to absorb Na$^+$ and passive mechanisms to absorb Na$^+$, Cl$^-$, and H$_2$O. In cholera, massive secretion of Cl$^-$ occurs, which draws Na$^+$ and H$_2$O into the gut lumen to produce a torrential secretory diarrhea. Effective treatment of choleraic diarrhea involves instillation of a glucose-Na$^+$ solution to activate the cotransporter, which also enhances passive absorption of Cl$^-$ and H$_2$O, thereby overriding the effects of Cl$^-$ secretion.

could have been given to simply treating at this stage (as would have been recommended if the diarrhea had occurred while traveling), rather than ordering a multitude of tests. Tests for HIV-associated or unusual organisms would only have been relevant if the diarrhea had persisted and routine cultures were negative.

Treatment must address prompt oral rehydration, as well as specific therapy to shorten the course of continued diarrhea. Oral rehydration formulas are available and can be obtained in foreign countries, but in the United States, agents such as Pedialyte or Gatorade are good alternatives. Ideally, 4 to 5 L should be consumed during the first 24 hr.

Specific treatments include bismuth subsalicylate (Pepto-Bismol), loperamide, or antibiotics (doxycycline, trimethoprim-sulfamethoxazole, ciprofloxacin), all of which will shorten the duration of illness.

With oral rehydration, loperamide, and doxycycline, this patient's diarrhea stopped in 24 hr. He was able to return to a normal diet with no recurrence of diarrhea.

CLINICAL OVERVIEW

Oral rehydration with glucose-electrolyte solutions remains the foundation for treatment of secretory diarrheas of any origin; intravenous fluids should be reserved for patients who are vomiting or are severely volume depleted. In any patient suffering acute infectious diarrhea, the major initial objective is fluid and electrolyte resuscitation for the following reasons. First, the major acute, serious complications of infectious diarrheas are dehydration and electrolyte abnormalities, which in extreme cases can evolve into circulatory shock and death. Second, the direct infectious complications of the intestinal infection are rarely emergent or initially overwhelming. Finally, more than 95% of acute infectious diarrheas resolve without direct treatment of the infection per se. Treatment of the intestinal infection is valuable only because this may shorten the period of diarrhea and volume depletion.

Nevertheless, infectious diarrheal disease remains one of the most lethal illnesses worldwide because of the inaccessibility of appropriate rehydration treatment to populations in underdeveloped nations. During the twentieth century, the major medical advance in the management of severe infectious diarrhea has been the clinical application of laboratory research. This research showed that instillation of glucose-containing electrolyte solutions into the upper gut promulgated intestinal absorption of fluid, even in the presence of a "torrential diarrhea" such as that in cholera (see Fig. 4–11).

CHAPTER FIVE

Digestion and Absorption of Carbohydrates and Proteins

CASE REPORT: INITIAL INFORMATION

A 27-year-old woman was referred to your office for lactose intolerance that did not respond to a restricted lactose intake. The patient had been in good health until 1 year previously, when she developed abdominal cramps, bloating, watery diarrhea, and flatulence. Typically, her symptoms began in the early afternoon, increased in intensity through the remainder of the day, and were gone by the next morning. She would have four or five watery, nonbloody, nongreasy bowel movements each day, with only rare nocturnal diarrhea. Before the onset of the present illness, her normal bowel habit had been two semiformed bowel movements per day. The patient denied foreign travel, drinking unprocessed water, risk factors for human immunodeficiency virus (HIV), or the use of medications, including antibiotics.

Previously the patient had presented to her doctor after 1 month of symptoms and a decrease in weight from 130 to 125 lb. At that time her physical examination was reported as normal, as was a complete blood cell count and a biochemical profile. Stool examinations for white cells, culture, ova, and parasites were negative. Her typical dietary intake included bran cereal, orange juice, and a glass of milk for breakfast; a sandwich or salad with a nondiet soft drink for lunch; and a meat and starch with milk or a soft drink for dinner. Her physician wondered whether the patient might have lactose or fructose intolerance, and he stopped all milk products and soft drinks sweetened with fructose. On returning 2 weeks later, the patient reported feeling 80% better, with two or three formed bowel movements a day, less cramping and flatulence, and stable weight. A recurrence of severe symptoms with a challenge of two glasses of milk confirmed the impression of lactose intolerance. The physician explained carbohydrate malabsorption to the patient and asked her to return if new problem ensued.

Ten months later the patient returned to her doctor, globally not feeling well. Despite rigorously maintaining her dietary lactose and fructose exclusions, she was having two or three loose bowel movements per day, her weight had decreased to 112 lb, flatulence and bloating persisted, and she was quite fatigued. Physical examination revealed a thin woman with mild pretibial edema, no blood in the stool, and no other abnormal findings. Repeated laboratory tests revealed a mild normochromic, normocytic anemia, a serum albumin level of 2.6 gm/dl, and a low serum iron level and iron-binding capacity. Thyroid function tests, stool cultures for ova and parasites, urinalysis, and liver biochemistry tests were normal. The patient was then referred to you for further evaluation. You find the physical examination to be identical to that noted previously.

PHYSIOLOGY

This section describes the mechanisms by which the small intestine handles two vital classes of nutrients: carbohydrates and proteins. Some generalizations are worth noting before considering the specific details of events involved in the assimilation of each class of nutrients:

1. Most, if not all of the digestion and absorption of these dietary nutrients occurs in the upper half of the small intestine.
2. Digestion of carbohydrates and proteins involves a series of physical and chemical alterations that make the nutrient molecules more soluble in water and facilitate their binding to transporters on the microvillus membrane of the enterocyte. For carbohydrates and proteins, digestion also involves enzymatic conversion of larger molecules into smaller molecules. The events of digestion are a necessary prelude, without which normal absorption will not occur.
3. Absorption of these nutrients is primarily via transcellular transport during the postprandial period and is a complex activity that requires initial binding to receptors located on the apical membrane of enterocytes. Subsequently, the absorptive process continues inside the enterocyte and involves diffusion across the cytosol and basolateral membrane into the interstitium.
4. Transcellular transport of the digestion products of dietary carbohydrate and protein is dominated by a positive feedback mechanism. This mechanism is the critical need of the upper gut to absorb all of the digested nutrients in a rapid fashion to ensure assimilation of 100% of the ingested protein and most of the digestible carbohydrate.

Intestinal Handling of Carbohydrates

Carbohydrates are the most important element of the diet from a caloric viewpoint. Worldwide, most people obtain more than half of their total caloric intake from carbohydrates, and carbohydrates are the cheapest dietary source of energy. The average American adult consumes about 300 gm of carbohydrates each day. The U.S. government has recommended that Americans increase the proportion of carbohydrates consumed daily.

Dietary carbohydrates consist of both digestible and indigestible carbohydrates. Digestible carbohydrates include the following:

- Starch (complex polysaccharide found in potato, flour, rice, etc.); this constitutes half of the ingested carbohydrates in the United States.
- Sucrose (table sugar); this constitutes 30% of the ingested carbohydrates in the United States.
- Fructose (from fruits).
- Lactose (from milk and milk products); this is nonessential for adult nutrition but is critical in infant and child nutrition.

Indigestible carbohydrate (the major component of dietary fiber) primarily consists of cellulose from vegetables.

Digestion of Carbohydrates

Dietary carbohydrates are mostly either disaccharides (a complex of two sugar molecules) or longer chains of sugar molecules. The intestine will absorb only single sugar molecules (e.g., glucose, galactose, fructose), and thus the more complex dietary carbohydrates have to be digested into single sugar molecules.

Digestion of starch involves two stages, one in the lumen and one in the microvilli (Fig. 5–1). In the initial stage, starch is digested into smaller molecules that require additional decomposition before they can be absorbed.

Starches are complex sugars that consist of long chains of glucose molecules with side branches of glucose. The main chain sugars are linked to one another by an alpha-1,4 glucosidic bond, whereas each side branch is connected to the main chain by a single alpha-1,6 glucosidic bond (Fig. 5–2). The enzyme alpha-amylase is secreted by the salivary glands and the pancreas. Alpha-amylase breaks the alpha 1,4 bonds between glucose molecules in the main chain and in the branch chain, except for the 1,4 bond at either end of a chain. Therefore, alpha-amylase in the lumen of the mouth, stomach, and small intestine converts starch into three major, but smaller, subunits, namely:

1. Alpha-limit dextrins (a main chain of two or three glucose molecules connected to a side chain of two or three glucose molecules by an alpha-1,6 bond);
2. Maltotriose (three glucose molecules connected by alpha-1,4 bonds); and
3. Maltose (two glucose molecules connected by an alpha-1,4 bond).

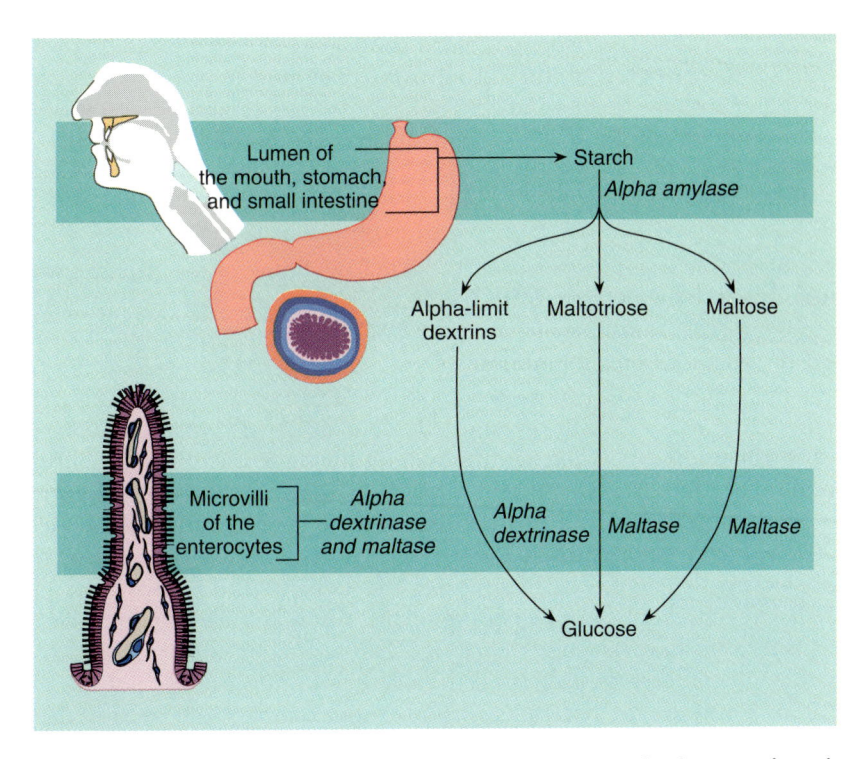

FIGURE 5–1. Digestion of starch involves two stages: one in the gastrointestinal lumen and the other in the microvilli of enterocytes. In the mouth, stomach, and intestinal lumen, starch is degraded by alpha-amylase into dextrin, maltotriose, and maltose. Disaccharidase enzymes in the microvilli further digest the starch degradation products into glucose.

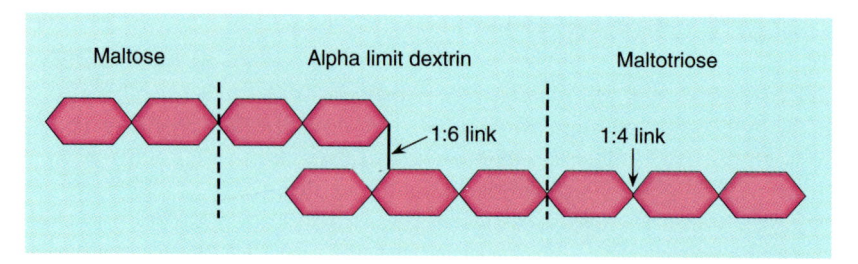

FIGURE 5–2. Digestion products of starch. Alpha-amylase splits the long-chain starch molecule at the 1:4 glucosidic linkages, except at either end of the chain, thereby digesting starch into maltotriose and maltose molecules. Alpha-amylase cannot split the 1:6 glucosidic linkages, which results in the production of alpha-limit dextrins from the side chains.

These three products of starch digestion reach the microvilli of the enterocyte, which contain disaccharidases. The disaccharidases break the starch digestion products into unattached glucose molecules:

$$\text{alpha-limit dextrin} \xrightarrow{\text{alpha-dextrinase}} \text{maltotriose, maltose, and glucose molecules}$$

$$\text{maltotriose} \xrightarrow{\text{maltase}} \text{three glucose molecules}$$

$$\text{maltose} \xrightarrow{\text{maltase}} \text{two glucose molecules}$$

Once in the form of glucose, the carbohydrate can bind to its transporter and be absorbed into the enterocyte. Inside the cell, glucose diffuses to and crosses the basolateral membrane into the interstitial space and finally into the blood.

Sucrose (simple table sugar) is digested by sucrase to form glucose and fructose:

$$\text{sucrose} \xrightarrow{\text{sucrase}} \text{glucose + fructose}$$

The sweetness of table sugar comes from the fructose. Some of the fructose will be used by the enterocyte as a fuel source.

Lactose is a dietary disaccharide composed of glucose and galactose; it is split by lactase located in the microvillus membrane.

$$\text{lactose} \xrightarrow{\text{lactase}} \text{glucose + galactose}$$

Galactose and glucose compete for binding sites on the same microvillus membrane transport molecule.

Some adults experience cramping and diarrhea after ingesting milk, which is not a major health concern, because milk is not essential in the adult diet. These individuals may have a lactase deficiency. In many cases the deficiency develops after childhood. Roughly 30% of white adults are lactase deficient, whereas 75% of adult blacks, Asians, and Native Americans have a lactase deficiency. The prevalence of symptoms from lactase deficiency depends on diet, as well as on the prevalence and intensity of the defect. For example, Asian adults do not generally consume milk or milk products, and they have no symptoms, despite a very high rate of lactase deficiency. By contrast, only 3% of Danes are deficient in lactase (as compared with 97% of Thais), and the Danish diet is very high in milk products.

Lactase deficiency in infants and young children can be much more serious. Infants depend on milk exclusively until their weaning or introduction to solid food. In lactase deficiency (Fig. 5–3), milk sugar (lactose) is ingested and reaches the upper small intestine, where no lactase is present. Hence, there is no splitting of lactose, and this undigested carbohydrate is propelled along the intestine, where it constitutes an overload of solute, thereby causing osmotic movement of water into the lumen of the small intestine. The result is osmotic diarrhea. Lactose is propelled into the colon to be metabolized into lactic acid by bacteria that can utilize lactose as a fuel source. This causes an increase in H^+ concentration in the lumen of the colon and a decrease in sodium absorption, which further aggravates the diarrhea (see Chapter 4). The bacteria utilizing lactose give off CO_2 as a metabolic product, and this gas distends the colon and causes pain to the infant. The infant does not get enough calories and, therefore, loses weight, cries constantly, and is always hungry. The treatment is to provide alternative sources of carbohydrate in the infant's diet. Formulas are available that substitute fructose for lactose. Beef broth is also a good substitute for the protein of milk.

Even in normal individuals without known disaccharidase deficiencies, some of the ingested wheat starch is not digested and reaches the colon as such. Anaerobic colonic bacteria metabolize this carbohydrate into short-chain fatty acids, such as butyrate, which can be absorbed from the colon. Butyrate is also a substrate for bacterial formation of flatus.

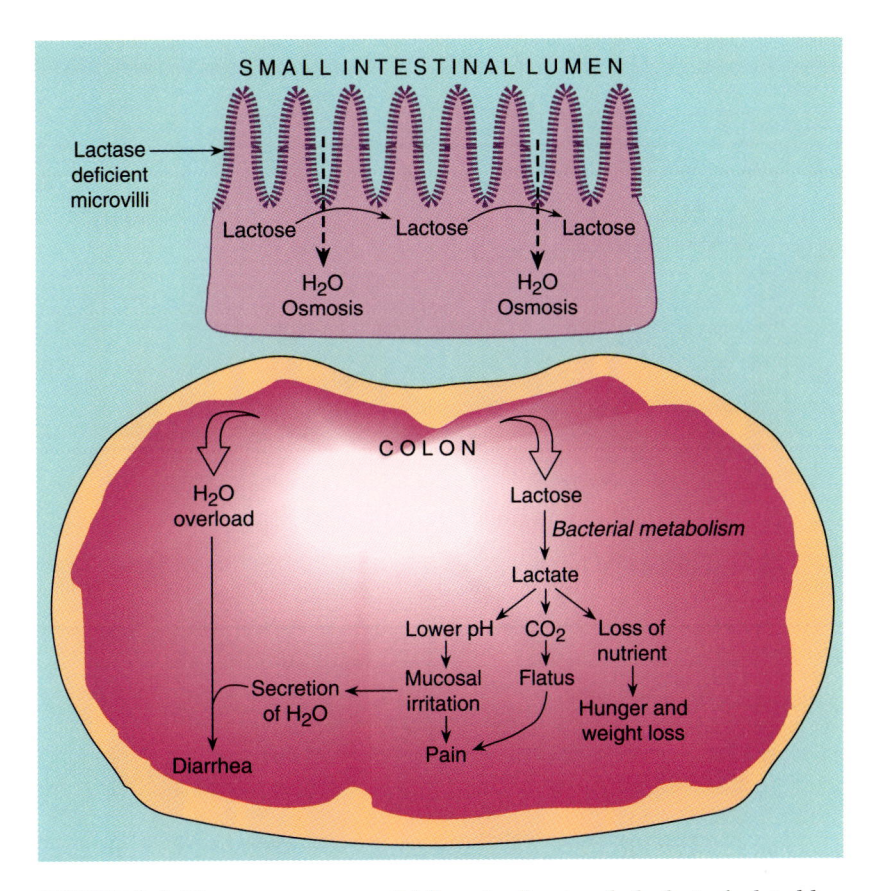

FIGURE 5–3. The consequences of failure to digest carbohydrate: isolated lactase deficiency. In the small bowel, solute excess and intraluminal secretion of water overwhelm normal absorptive functions. The result is diarrhea, abdominal pain, and loss of nutrient calories.

Absorption of Carbohydrates

There is considerable evidence that glucose is absorbed by active (energy-dependent) transport mechanisms. Thus, if glucose concentration is higher in blood than in the gut lumen, glucose will not remain in the lumen. Instead, it will be absorbed from the lumen against its concentration gradient. Furthermore, if the concentration of glucose in the blood is equal to the concentration in the lumen, no net movement of glucose would be expected if it were only passively transported; nevertheless, there is a net movement of glucose from the lumen into the blood. This movement of glucose against a concentration gradient from the intestinal lumen into the blood requires the expenditure of energy. In addition, Na^+ must be in the lumen for glucose to be absorbed, and Na^+ is actively transported by enterocytes. Poisons that block energy metabolism (e.g., cyanide) stop the net entry of glucose into the blood when the concentration of glucose is lower in the lumen than in the blood. The efficiency of the active glucose transport system is very high. Normally all dietary glucose available in the lumen is absorbed.

Glucose absorption is facilitated by the active cotransport of Na^+ (Fig. 5–4). Glucose and Na^+ in the intestinal lumen bind to a transporter on the apical surface of the ente-

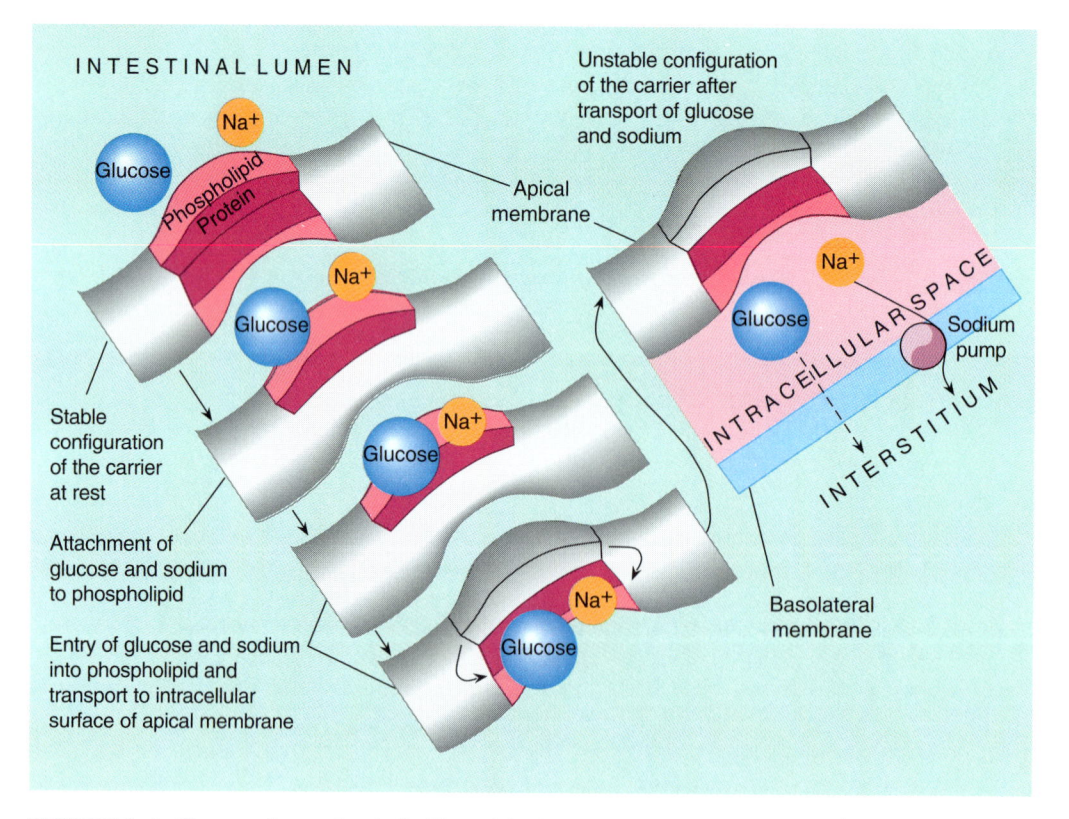

FIGURE 5–4. Glucose absorption is facilitated by its active cotransport with Na^+. This cotransport involves binding and uptake of both glucose and Na^+ to the phospholipid portion of the transporter, a change in transporter configuration caused by movement of the protein portion of the transporter, and release of glucose and Na^+ into the cytosol of the enterocyte. Glucose diffuses out of the cell into the interstitium. Na^+ is actively pumped out of the cell.

rocyte when the transporter is in its stable configuration. The transporter has two components: a phospholipid, which serves as the binding site for glucose and Na^+, and a protein, which is the mobile part of the complex. Glucose and Na^+ enter the phospholipid portion, which causes the protein portion of the transporter to undergo a conformational change and flip inward. This movement transports glucose and Na^+ into the intracellular space of the enterocyte.

At this point, glucose is present in high concentrations in the cytosol, so it will passively diffuse into the interstitial space and then into the blood to be circulated to the tissues. Na^+ is actively pumped from the intracellular space across the basolateral membranes into the interstitium by the sodium pump, Na^+,K^+-ATPase. The entire process is driven by the sodium pump, which maintains a concentration gradient for Na^+ such that the movement of Na^+ is favored from the intestinal lumen into the intracellular space. Glucose is linked to Na^+ movement and is co-transported from the lumen into the enterocyte. The presence of glucose in the lumen also increases absorption of Na^+ from the gut, an important mechanism utilized in the treatment of cholera (see Chapter 4). Any glucose that diffuses from the intracellular space back into the lumen is taken up by the transporter again and placed back into the intracellular space. Thus, the transporter acts as a barrier to passive glucose movement back into the intestinal lumen.

Galactose also binds to the same transporter as glucose but has a lower affinity for the transporter than does glucose. Glucose will be transported more avidly by the carrier than galactose; thus, in an equimolar solution of both sugars, glucose will be absorbed faster than galactose. However, if the glucose concentration is low and the galactose concentration is sufficiently high, galactose can competitively inhibit glucose uptake.

Fructose is passively absorbed into the enterocyte. The enterocyte can use fructose to generate ATP for its cellular activities by phosphorylating this sugar into fructose-6-phosphate. As the fructose is used up in the enterocyte or diffuses from the cell into the blood, there will be a low intracellular concentration compared with the fructose concentration in the lumen of the gut, and fructose will continue to be absorbed passively into the enterocyte.

Intestinal Handling of Proteins

Proteins are the "expensive" food in the diet. Meat, fish, eggs, and dairy products are rich sources of protein. In most underdeveloped countries, inexpensive vegetables are the main source of protein but are a much poorer source of this key nutrient than is meat. An American adult requires 50 gm of protein in the diet each day to maintain nitrogen balance. In underdeveloped countries, there is an increased risk of protein deficiency because of a borderline intake of protein. Kwashiorkor, which causes edema, ascites, and fatty liver, is common in the tropics among children subsisting on a diet marginally adequate in calories but grossly deficient in protein. In the United States, where meat is readily available and relatively inexpensive, protein, on the average, constitutes about 25% of the total caloric intake.

Protein must be digested before it can be absorbed. Pepsin, trypsin, and carboxypeptidase metabolize dietary proteins into tripeptides, dipeptides, and amino acids, all of which can be absorbed. Therefore, essentially 100% of the protein ingested is absorbed.

Protein is needed to compensate for constant protein breakdown and loss from the body. The gut also contributes to the protein loss. Sources of fecal protein loss from the intestine include the following:

- bacteria,
- sloughed cells from the epithelial lining of the gut (every 3 days, about half of the intestinal lining is shed), and
- secretory products from goblet cells (mucin, polypeptides).

Devastating chronic illnesses (e.g., cancer, heart failure, tuberculosis) can lead to a wasting condition as a result of loss of appetite. In a wasting condition, the body loses not only total weight but also muscle mass.

Digestion of Proteins

As is the case with starch, the digestion of proteins occurs in two stages (Fig. 5–5). In the lumen of the stomach and intestine, endopeptidases (pepsin, trypsin) cleave internal peptide bonds, and exopeptidases (carboxypeptidases) cleave C-terminal amino acids from the protein molecule. These enzymes break down ingested proteins into tripeptides and dipeptides, which can be absorbed as such, and into amino acids, which can also be absorbed. At the microvillus membrane of the enterocyte, some tripeptides and dipeptides are cleaved further by membrane-bound proteases into amino acids.

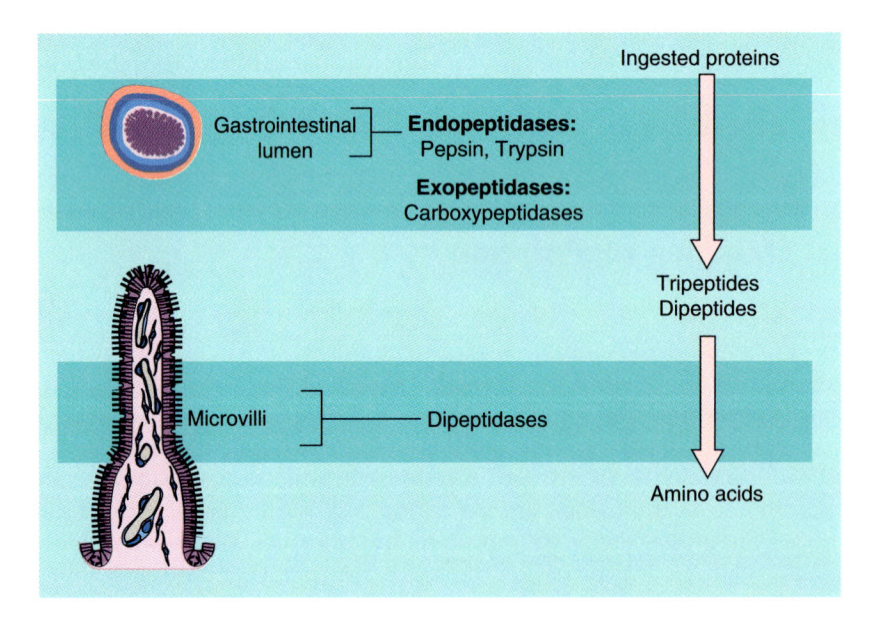

FIGURE 5–5. Digestion of proteins involves two stages: one in the gastrointestinal lumen and the other in the microvilli of enterocytes. Protein is degraded into smaller molecules (i.e., polypeptides, tripeptides, dipeptides, and amino acids) by pepsin in the stomach and by pancreatic trypsin and carboxypeptidase in the intestinal lumen. Dipeptidases in the microvillus membrane digest tripeptides and dipeptides into amino acids. All ingested protein is digested into amino acids (75%), dipeptides, and tripeptides, all of which are absorbed.

Absorption of Protein Digestion Products

Amino acids are rapidly absorbed into the intracellular space. Furthermore, active cotransport of amino acids with Na^+ ensures that all dietary protein will be absorbed. About 75% of dietary protein is digested into amino acids and absorbed in that form; the other 25% is absorbed as dipeptides and tripeptides. The process of amino acid (AA) absorption is similar to glucose cotransport with Na^+:

$$AA + Na^+ \text{ in the lumen} \xrightarrow{transporter} Na^+ \text{ in intracellular space} \xrightarrow{pump} \text{interstitial space}$$

$$AA \text{ in intracellular space} \xrightarrow{diffusion} \text{interstitial space}$$

There are four separate types of transporters for different groups of AAs (Fig. 5–6). Each type of transporter will bind and transport certain AAs only. Thus, the transporter for dibasic AAs will not transport neutral AAs, and the transporter for dicarboxylic AAs will not transport a special AA such as glycine. Within each group of AAs, all the characteristics of a transporter-facilitated process are present (e.g., saturation, competitive inhibition).

Patients with Hartnup's disease display multiple disorders in the absorption of tryptophane. In Hartnup's disease, an autosomal recessive metabolic disorder exists that is characterized by an aminoaciduria. The carrier system for neutral AAs is absent, so the neonate cannot absorb tryptophane from the lumen of the small intestine or the renal tubule. Because the nephron will not reabsorb tryptophane, which has been filtered by the glomerulus, tryptophane appears in the urine. Tryptophane deficiency results in cerebellar ataxia and a light-sensitive skin rash. However, some tripeptides and dipeptides that contain tryptophane are absorbed from the small intestine, and tryptophane, if linked to another amino acid, may be able to enter the intracellular space of the enterocyte. This source of tryptophane makes its way to the blood and subsequently to the tissues.

Hartnup's disease can be detected in some cases by a unique finding. The tryptophane that is not absorbed from the small intestine passes through to the colon, where bacteria convert tryptophane to indican. Indican is absorbed from the colon, diffuses into the blood, and travels to the kidney to be filtered. In its diseased state, the nephron is not capable of reabsorbing indican, so indican is also excreted into the urine. Once in the urine, indican reacts with Cl^- and turns the urine blue in color. Hence, this condition is also known as the blue diaper syndrome.

FIGURE 5–6. Active transport systems for amino acids consist of four types. Each type is specific for one group of amino acids and will not transport amino acids outside that group. There is competition for transport binding sites between members of one group of amino acids, and saturation of binding sites can occur if the concentration of amino acids becomes too high.

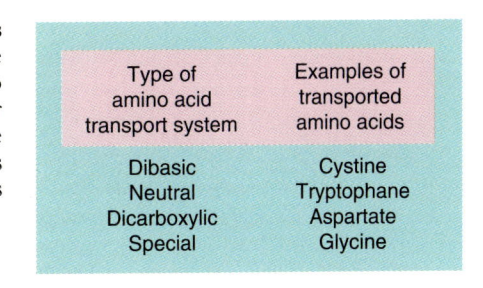

Type of amino acid transport system	Examples of transported amino acids
Dibasic	Cystine
Neutral	Tryptophane
Dicarboxylic	Aspartate
Special	Glycine

CASE REPORT: CONCLUSION

CLINICAL IMPRESSION. The patient's clinical course was most compatible with a small intestinal disease causing malabsorption. Primary lactose intolerance was a reasonable diagnosis to exclude at the onset of illness, but the continued weight loss with bloating, edema, and hypoalbuminemia suggested that the lactose intolerance may have been secondary to a mucosal disease that was not primary or genetic. Demonstration of malabsorption depended on measuring fat in the stool and absorption of D-xylose, and therefore, these tests were performed. The excretion of fat in the stool was 11 gm/day (normal, ≤6 gm/day), and D-xylose absorption was 50% of normal. These findings were compatible with either a diffuse mucosal disease, such as celiac sprue, or a partial small bowel obstruction, perhaps caused by ileitis with bacterial overgrowth. Therefore, a small bowel biopsy or a small bowel radiograph would be justified at this time, and the biopsy was performed.

Small bowel biopsy specimens demonstrated total villus atrophy compatible with celiac sprue. The patient was placed on a strict gluten exclusion diet. In 4 weeks, the patient had no diarrhea or bloating, had gained 10 lb, had no edema, and had a serum albumin concentration of 3.4 gm/dl.

CLINICAL OVERVIEW

Effective management of a patient with malabsorption syndrome depends on making a specific causal diagnosis. Knowing the etiology of the malabsorption provides an advantage that cannot be replaced by therapeutic trials or treatment with a broad range of nutritional supplements. Such therapeutic approaches should be relegated to the rare case of malabsorption syndrome in which the cause cannot be determined.

The patient suffering malabsorption syndrome may present with unusual features, and the diagnosis requires a high degree of clinical suspicion. For example, on initial presentation, the patient may not have experienced diarrhea or weight loss, and thus the first problem revealed may be a mixed anemia that has developed because of proximal small bowel malabsorption of folate and iron. Other atypical presenting problems may include osteomalacia, osteopenia, and elevated alkaline phosphatase levels from malabsorption of Ca^{++} and vitamin D; hypoalbuminemia and muscle wasting from malabsorption of protein or associated enteropathy causing protein loss; and night blindness or bleeding dyscrasias caused by malabsorption of vitamin A or vitamin K.

The diagnostic approach to malabsorption syndrome requires documentation of malabsorption with quantifiable laboratory tests—namely, the measurement of fecal fat (>6 gm/day constitutes steatorrhea) and the oral D-xylose test. If the result of both tests are abnormal, malabsorption rather than maldigestion is the presumptive diagnosis. If the D-xylose test result is normal despite quantified steatorrhea, the underlying process is probably maldigestion (e.g., pancreatic exocrine insufficiency). The next diagnostic test should be a small bowel biopsy, which should define the cause of malabsorption. The most prevalent causes of intestinal malabsorption that can be positively identified from a mucosal biopsy of the small bowel include celiac sprue, Whipple's disease, lymphangiectasia, lymphoma, hypogammaglobulinemia, and parasitic disease (giardiasis). Other causes of intestinal malabsorption in which the mucosal biopsy will probably be normal or nondiagnostic include Zollinger-Ellison syndrome, laxative abuse, short bowel syndrome, bacterial overgrowth, and HIV infection. Definitive diagnosis of any one of these will require positive findings from other laboratory tests.

CHAPTER SIX

Digestion and Absorption of Lipids

CASE REPORT: INITIAL INFORMATION

A 67-year-old man was referred from the emergency room for your evaluation of his abdominal pain, diarrhea, and weight loss of 3 months duration. The patient had been in his usual state of health until 3 months previously, when he developed gradually worsening abdominal pain. The pain was in the midepigastrium and radiated through to the back. Ten years earlier a similar pain had been ascribed to an ulcer and had remitted after a month's treatment with a bland diet and cimetidine. This pain occurred at any time of the day, lasted for 2 to 3 hr, increased after eating, and was not affected by antacids. The patient had lost 14 lb in the preceding 3 months. Two months earlier he had begun having four to five semiformed bowel movements per day. The movements had a greasy appearance and a foul odor but were without blood and melena. Two weeks before presentation, after what appeared to be trivial trauma, he had developed a large hematoma on his right buttock. Persisting symptoms led to his visit to the emergency room.

There were no significant past medical problems or operations other than the presumed ulcer 10 years previously. He was a 90-pack/year smoker and drank three to four beers each night. His wife had died of lung cancer 6 months before. There was no relevant family history.

Physical examination revealed a chronically ill–appearing man in mild distress. There was a large hematoma over the right buttock spreading down to the thigh. The conjunctivae were icteric. Examination of the abdomen revealed tenderness on palpation of the epigastrium with mild guarding and no rebound. There were no masses. Percussion revealed that the liver was 13 cm in span at the midclavicular line. The spleen was not palpated, the rectal examination was normal, and a Hemoccult test was negative. The patient had 2+ pitting edema to the knees but no evidence of ascites.

Initial laboratory tests were normal, with the following exceptions: Hct = 39%; prothrombin time = 15 sec (normal, <11 sec); aspartate aminotransferase (AST) = 124 U/L (normal, <35 U/L); alanine aminotransferase (ALT) = 197 U/L (normal, <40 U/L); bilirubin = 3.6 mg/dl (normal, <1.1 mg/dl); alkaline phosphatase = 1270 IU/ml (normal, <125 IU/ml); albumin = 2.1 gm/dl (normal, >3.6 gm/dl); and CA^{++} = 6.8 mg/dl (normal, >8.2 mg/dl). A chest radiograph demonstrated bullous emphysema without infiltration or evidence of masses.

PHYSIOLOGY

Triglycerides constitute about 98% of total dietary lipids. The remaining 2% consists of phospholipids and cholesterol. All three of these lipids are important constituents of all cell membranes. Cholesterol is the source material for the synthesis of steroid hormones and bile acids in the body; triglycerides provide essential fatty acids.

On oxidation in the tissues, fats provide more than twice as much energy per gram as carbohydrates. Fats also have a greater satiety value than carbohydrates, because they tend to remain in the stomach longer and are digested more slowly.

Digestion of Lipids

Ten percent of the dietary fat is hydrolyzed into glycerol and fatty acids by lipases secreted by the salivary and gastric glands in the mouth and stomach. Most dietary fat is digested in the upper small intestine, where special mechanisms have evolved to overcome two factors:

1. Dietary fats are not water soluble, and the lumen of the small intestine contains an aqueous medium.
2. Digestive enzymes for dietary lipids are dissolved in water and cannot effectively break down fat, unless the fat can be solubilized.

These difficulties in digesting fat in the gut are handled in two ways. First, fat is emulsified by bile salts and lipid digestion products (fatty acids, monoglycerides, and lysolecithin). Second, emulsified fat combines with bile salts to form micelles. The churning and mixing of food in the distal stomach breaks lipids into small droplets that are kept from coalescing by bile salts, lipid digestion products, and some dietary proteins.

Bile salts are complex molecules that can dissolve in both aqueous and lipid phases, thereby solubilizing (emulsifying) the lipid. Lipid digestion products and some dietary proteins have the same properties as bile salts in emulsifying dietary fat in an aqueous medium. The combination of bile salts and lipid digestion products completely emulsifies all dietary fat in the upper small intestine.

After emulsification, fat globules have an average diameter of 1000 Å. Bile salts then form micelles with lipid, thereby reducing the diameter of the bile salt–lipid complex to about 50 Å. This reduction of particle size increases the total surface area for enzyme activity by 20-fold.

Micelles consist of bile salts that completely surround a globule of digested dietary triglycerides in the lumen of the gut. The conjugated, squalene nuclear portion of the bile salt is directed into the fat globule, and the charged amino acid portion (taurine, glycine) is directed out into the aqueous environment. The uncharged hydrophobic tails of the bile salt molecules (i.e., the squalene nucleus) are packed in the micellar interior along with the hydrophobic tails of fatty acids, 2-monoglyceride, lysolecithin, cholesterol, and fat-soluble vitamins.

Thus, after a fatty meal, a sample of fluid from the small intestine will consist of two phases. The upper phase contains small globules of emulsified fat that are visible under bright light. The lower phase is totally clear but contains some lipid digestion products (fatty acids, cholesterol, monoglycerides) that have formed micelles with bile salts.

Lipase and Colipase

The pancreatic enzyme lipase B has an electrically negative charge, as do bile salts. Their mutual repulsion is prevented by a polypeptide cofactor, colipase, which is found in pancreatic juice and complexes lipase to bile salts at the surface of micelles (Fig. 6–1). Colipase also lowers the pH optimum for lipase activity to near the prevailing pH (6 to 7) found in the intestinal lumen. Thus, colipase acts as an anchor for lipase, allowing the enzyme to digest triglycerides. In addition, colipase also binds micelles, keeping them close to the site where lipase hydrolyzes triglycerides into monoglycerides and fatty acids. These digestion products are two of the major components of micelles in the gut.

Lipase can digest triglycerides into free fatty acids and 2-monoglyceride, which are much more soluble in bile salt micelles than are triglycerides. Lipolytic products also have a larger number of exposed hydrophilic groups than do triglycerides. This shift in degree of charge orientation results in greater solubility in water (Fig. 6–2).

Most dietary triglycerides come from meat, fish, and dairy products. The largest fraction of ingested lipid consists of long-chain fatty acids (C_{16}, C_{18}, C_{20}). Triglycerides from dairy sources consist of short- and medium-chain fatty acids (C_{12} or less), which are more soluble in water, and thus are easier to digest than are long-chain fatty acids. Dietary lipids, except for short- and medium-chain triglycerides and glycerol, require bile salts

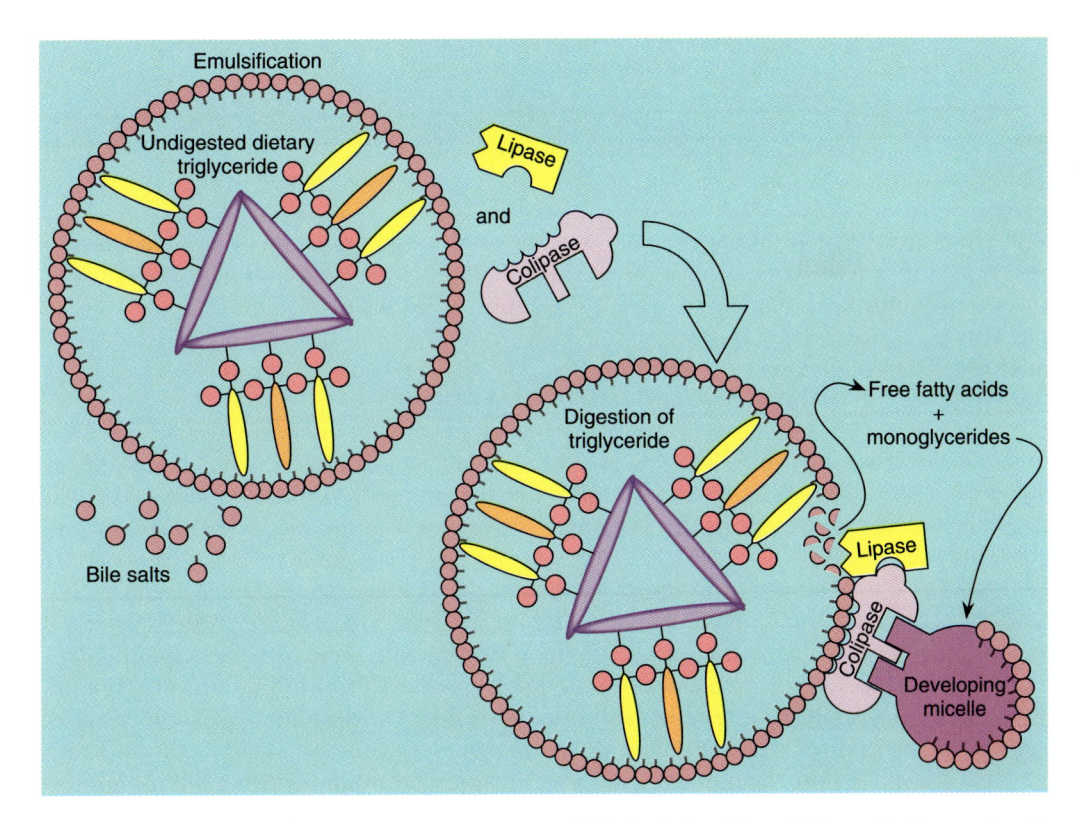

FIGURE 6–1. Colipase allows lipase to digest emulsified triglycerides. Colipase facilitates the digestion of lipid particles by pancreatic lipase in the gut lumen by complexing the enzyme to bile salts on the surface of the droplet of emulsified triglyceride. Colipase also binds micelles, allowing the entry of lipid digestion products into micelles.

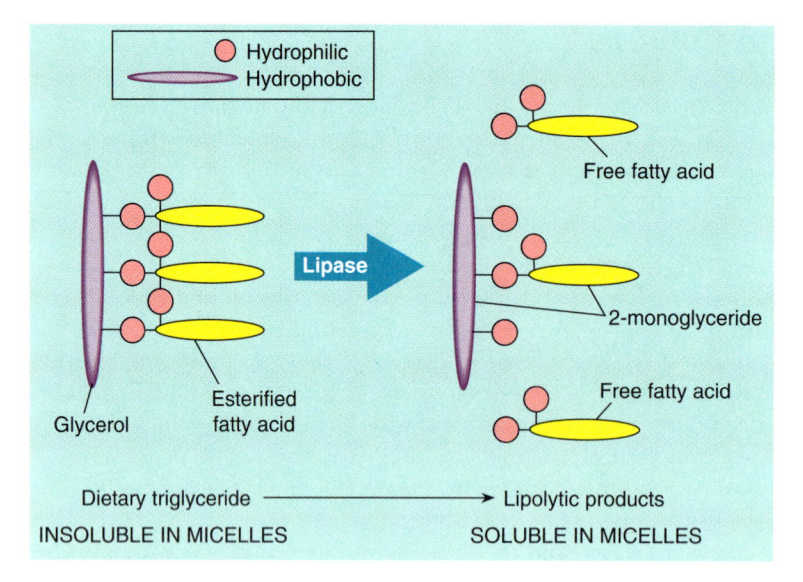

FIGURE 6–2. Lipase digests dietary lipid into products that are more soluble in bile acid micelles. Dietary triglycerides are insoluble in an aqueous medium, because most of their hydrophilic components are shielded from the polarized portions of water molecules. Digestion of the triglyceride into fatty acids and 2-monoglyceride produces smaller molecules whose hydrophilic portions are exposed to the charged parts of water molecules. These products can then be stacked in bile acid micelles with their hydrophobic portions in the center of the micelle and their hydrophilic components protruding into the aqueous medium.

and micelle formation for digestion and for absorption. Dietary lipids are hydrolyzed into lipid digestion products by three pancreatic enzymes: lipase, cholesterol ester hydrolase, and phospholipase A_2 (Fig. 6–3).

Absorption and Reconstruction of Lipids

Micelles transport lipid digestion products from the gut lumen to the microvilli of the enterocyte (Fig. 6–4). Micelles formed in the gut lumen each contain 1000 to 100,000 molecules of bile acids, fatty acids, 2-monoglyceride, lysolecithin, cholesterol, and fat-soluble vitamins.

Micelles diffuse into the unstirred layer adjacent to the enterocyte and then decompose, releasing their contents. The unstirred layer is acidic and protonates the fatty acids, making them less soluble in the micelle. Fatty acids, monoglycerides, lysolecithin, and cholesterol diffuse down their concentration gradients from the unstirred layer into the enterocyte. Bile acids in the unstirred layer diffuse down their concentration gradients back to the gut lumen, because they cannot enter the enterocytes of the proximal intestine. Eventually bile acids bind to receptors and are actively absorbed in the ileum of the intestine.

Micelles are stabilized by negative charges carried mainly by conjugated bile salt molecules. If the bile salt concentration is below 25 mmol/L (critical micellar concentration), micelles fail to form. The normal bile salt concentration in the intestine after a meal is approximately 40 mmol/L.

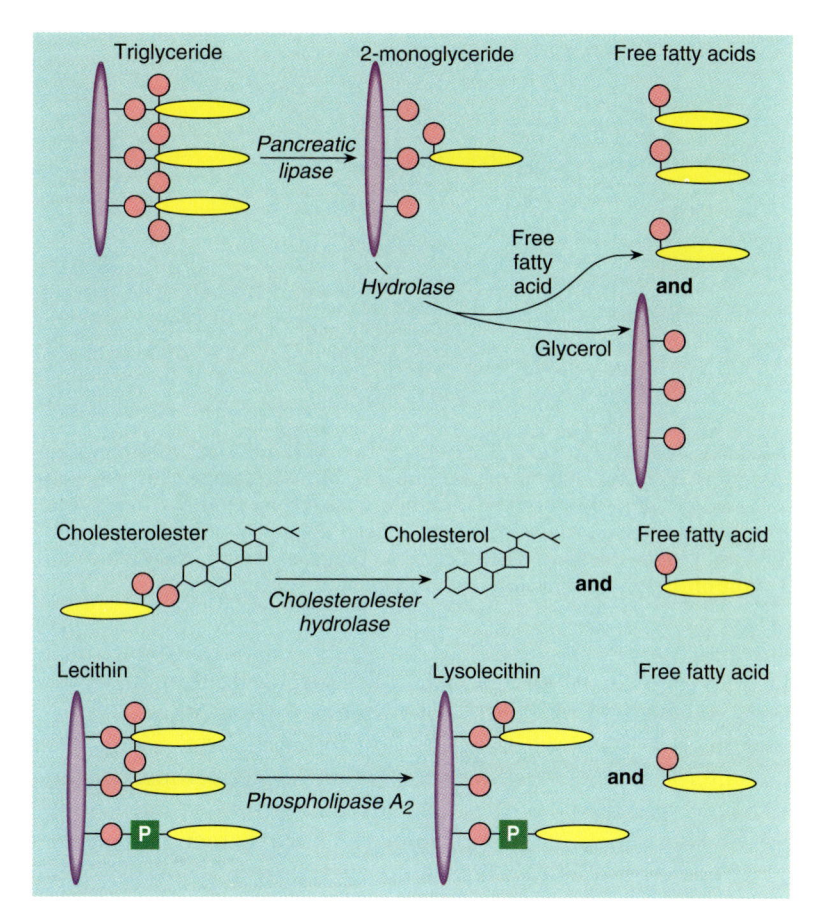

FIGURE 6–3. The three major dietary fats are digested into their respective digestion products by enzymes present in the proximal gut lumen. The large, insoluble dietary lipids are replaced mostly by smaller and more aqueous soluble fatty acids, monoglyceride, and glycerol. This conversion facilitates both emulsification and micelle formation.

The major lipid digestion products (free fatty acids and 2-monoglyceride) undergo reesterification inside the enterocyte to form new triglycerides (Fig. 6–5). The cytosol of the enterocyte contains fatty acid–binding proteins (FABP, Fig. 6–5), which have a high affinity for long-chain fatty acids. FABP transport long-chain fatty acids to the smooth endoplasmic reticulum of the enterocyte, where resynthesis of new triglycerides occurs. Fatty acids are activated to acyl-coenzyme A (acyl-CoA) in a reaction catalyzed by acyl-CoA synthetase. The reaction also involves coenzyme A, ATP, and Mg^{++}.

The next step in the resynthesis of new triglycerides is the conversion of monoglycerides (MG) into diglycerides (DG) and into triglycerides (TG):

$$\text{Acyl-CoA} + \text{monoglyceride} \xrightarrow{\text{MG transferase}} \text{diglyceride}$$
$$\text{Acyl-CoA} + \text{diglyceride} \xrightarrow{\text{DG transferase}} \text{triglyceride}$$

During fasting there is a second reaction that dominates resynthesis of TG: the phosphatidic acid pathway. In this reaction, acyl-CoA combines with alpha-glycerophosphate from

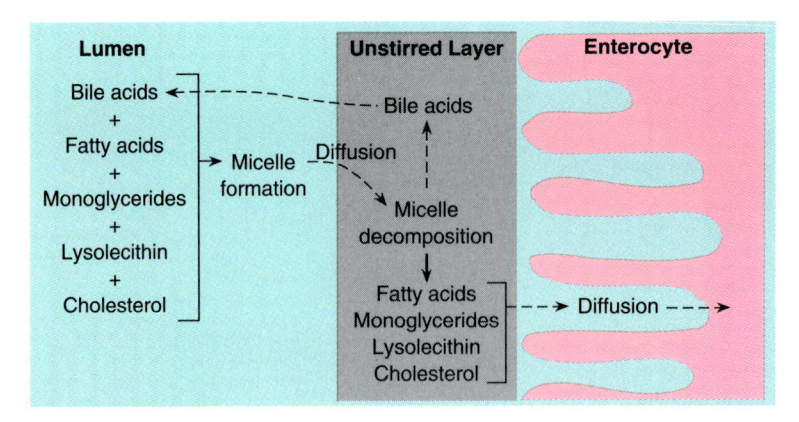

FIGURE 6–4. The micelle is a vehicle for movement of lipid digestion products from the lumen of the gut into the enterocyte. Micelles containing lipid digestion products and bile acids diffuse from the lumen into the unstirred layer, where the micelle decomposes. The high concentration of lipid-soluble materials adjacent to the enterocyte surface allows diffusion of these materials into the intracellular space.

glucose metabolism to form TG and phospholipids such as lecithin. Absorbed lysolecithin from micelles is also acylated inside the enterocyte to form lecithin.

After resynthesis of TG, lipid particles begin to form in the region of the Golgi apparatus of the enterocyte. These particles are called "chylomicrons." Chylomicrons consist mostly (90%) of reformed TG; the other lipids in chylomicrons include cholesterol, phospholipids, and beta-lipoprotein. A chylomicron has a diameter of 1000 Å, and its core contains TG and cholesterol. The surface of the chylomicron is covered by phospholipids and beta-lipoprotein, the latter being water-soluble, thereby allowing chylomicrons to emulsify. In the disorder abetalipoproteinemia, enterocytes are unable to form beta-lipoprotein, and chylomicrons cannot be transported out of the enterocyte. The result is malabsorption of fat.

After chylomicrons develop in the Golgi apparatus, they coalesce to form secretory vesicles, which migrate to the basolateral membrane of the enterocyte. The membrane of the secretory vesicle, containing chylomicrons, fuses with the enterocyte membrane, and the chylomicrons are secreted into the interstitium by the process of exocytosis. Chylomicrons then move through gaps between endothelial cells of the lymphatics and are carried off in the lymph flow, eventually reaching the systemic circulation by way of the thoracic duct. After a fatty meal, chylomicrons compose one tenth of the lymph. Some lipid digestion products do not reach the body via lymphatics but gain access via the bloodstream directly from the enterocyte; these include glycerol and short- and medium-chain fatty acids.

Intestinal Malabsorption of Fat

Intestinal malabsorption of lipids is caused by two main processes: failure to emulsify dietary fat and lack of an adequate mucosal absorptive surface. Failure to properly digest fat in the intestinal lumen occurs in pancreatitis, pancreatic carcinoma, and cystic fibrosis. In these disorders, pancreatic enzymes are not secreted into the gut. In other diseases (e.g., hepatitis and obstruction of the common bile ducts by gallstones), bile salts do not

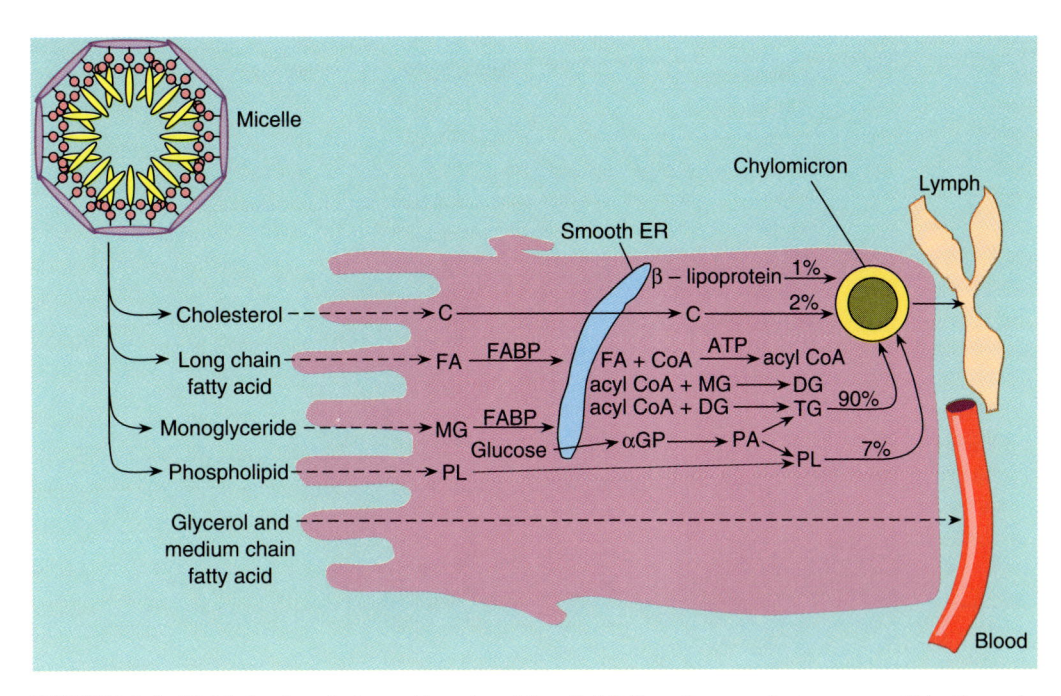

FIGURE 6–5. Multiple chemical reactions involving lipid digestion products occur within the enterocyte and reconstitute long-chain triglycerides for transport into lymphatics. Each of the micellar lipid digestion products becomes part of the synthetic process that forms chylomicrons, which contain mainly reconstituted long-chain triglycerides. The enterocyte then extrudes chylomicrons into the interstitium, from which these lipid structures diffuse into lymphatic capillaries. C = Cholesterol; FA = free fatty acid; MG = 2-monoglyceride; PL = phospholipid; FABP = fatty acid–binding proteins; αGP = alpha-glycerophosphate; PA = phosphatidic acid; ER = endoplasmic reticulum; DG = diglyceride; and TG = triglyceride.

reach the intestine. If pancreatic enzymes are not available, dietary fat is not digested, and the feces are loaded with triglycerides. If bile salts are not available, dietary fat is digested but not absorbed, and the feces are loaded with fatty acids and 2-monoglyceride.

Loss of normal intestinal mucosal absorptive function can result from different causes (Fig. 6–6). Thus, surgical resection or bypass of long segments of small bowel, especially the ileum; local mucosal reaction to drugs or toxins; or congenital deficiency of an enzyme (e.g., gluten hydrolase, which breaks down gluten) can evoke intestinal malabsorption. In these disorders the lipids are digested, but the mucosa is unable to transport normal quantities of fat.

Normally, almost all dietary fat is absorbed, and less than 6 gm/day is excreted in the feces. Stool fat is derived from sloughing of mucosal cells, from bacterial cell walls, and from colonic secretions, rather than from ingested fat. Measurement of fat content in feces is a clinical indicator of malabsorption syndromes. Steatorrhea is defined as fecal fat exceeding 6 gm/day in a patient with a normal dietary intake.

CASE REPORT: CONCLUSION

CLINICAL IMPRESSION. This jaundiced, 67-year-old man with severe weight loss, malabsorptive-type stools, abdominal pain, and marked elevation of alkaline phosphatase most likely had a tumor in the pancreatic head. Other possibilities included chronic pancreatitis, with a phlegmon or pseudocyst partially obstructing

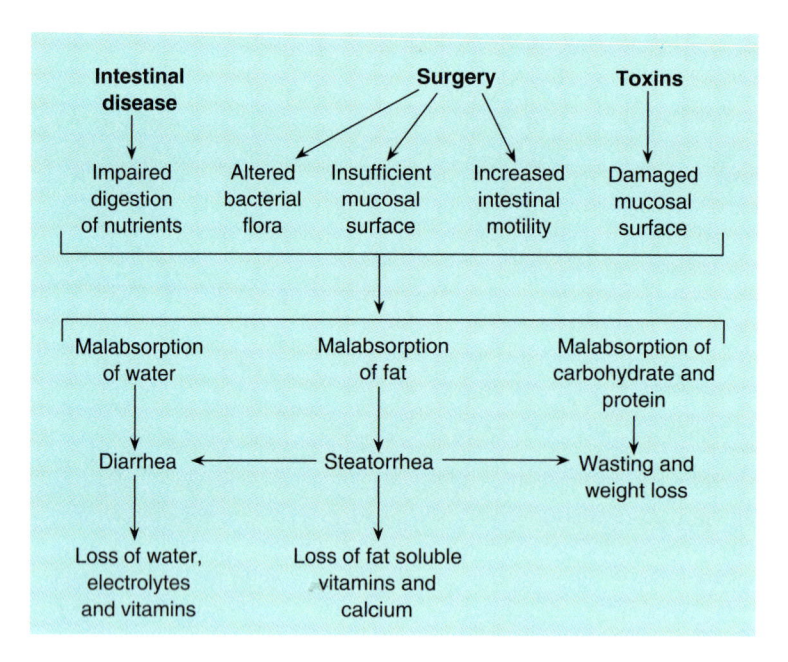

FIGURE 6–6. Intestinal malabsorption of lipids and other key nutrients occurs in many diseases that share one of two major deficits: impaired digestion of nutrients and insufficient mucosal surface available for transport. Once steatorrhea becomes established, it contributes to other malabsorptive problems, such as diarrhea; weight loss; and failure to adequately absorb Ca^{++} and vitamins A, D, E, and K.

the distal common bile duct, and a metastatic or primary tumor replacing most of the liver.

Parenteral vitamin K reverted the prothrombin time to normal. A computed tomographic (CT) scan of the abdomen revealed a 7-cm mass in the head of the pancreas, dilated extra- and intrahepatic bile ducts, and two 4-cm lucencies in the liver. Percutaneous biopsy specimens of the pancreatic mass and liver lesions revealed adenocarcinoma. The patient decided against additional diagnostic or therapeutic maneuvers, was placed on oral morphine, and was referred for home hospice care.

CLINICAL OVERVIEW

Maldigestion of fat and steatorrhea (>6 gm/day) are commonly found in patients with cancer of the head of the pancreas. When steatorrhea is documented in a patient with abdominal pain and jaundice, pancreatic head malignancy should be high on the differential diagnosis. Maldigestion of lipids with loss of caloric intake is responsible for dramatic weight losses in such a patient. By contrast, cancers of the body or tail of the pancreas do not cause steatorrhea, because pancreatic lipolytic enzyme secretion must be lowered 90% to develop steatorrhea. Because of their location, such malignancies are unlikely to obstruct the proximal main pancreatic duct, unlike cancer in the head of the pancreas.

In the case report, the patient's common bile duct was also obstructed by the pancreatic tumor, which caused jaundice and contributed to the steatorrhea; common bile duct obstruction alone rarely leads to significant steatorrhea. Once the mass was identified by CT scan, the differential diagnosis was between cancer of the head of the pancreas and chronic pancreatitis with a phlegmon obstructing the pancreatic and bile ducts. Chronic pancreatitis would be suggested by a long and constant history of attacks of prevertebral pain, which this patient did not have. A history of alcohol abuse is common in both pancreatitis and pancreatic cancer. With pancreatic cancer, metastases to the liver or bone are common. The positive laboratory finding of a markedly elevated level of CA-19-9 (an antigen that is elevated in numerous malignancies) in a patient with a pancreatic mass established by an imaging technique would also support the presumptive diagnosis of pancreatic carcinoma. However, definitive diagnosis requires histopathologic evidence from a percutaneous or operative biopsy specimen.

CHAPTER SEVEN

Mineral and Vitamin Absorption

CASE REPORT: INITIAL INFORMATION

A 42-year-old man with Crohn's disease moved to your city and wanted you to become his primary physician. He had been in his usual state of health until 8 years previously, when bloating and right lower quadrant abdominal pain began to occur 2 to 3 hr after most meals. Typically the pain would diminish after the patient had two or three loose but nonbloody bowel movements. He had lost 18 lb over a month's time and saw a physician. At that time he was afebrile, thin, and showed tenderness in the right lower quadrant. He had a normal hematocrit (Hct) with a white blood cell (WBC) count of 13,000, mild hypoalbuminemia, and an erythrocyte sedimentation rate of 60 mm/hr. Plain radiography of the abdomen demonstrated a mildly dilated small bowel with scattered air-fluid levels. On a small bowel series, the distal 13 cm of his ileum appeared narrowed and nodular, with some dilation of the otherwise normal small bowel proximal to the stricture. There were no fistulas.

These findings were thought to be compatible with Crohn's ileitis, and the patient was started on prednisone (30 mg) and sulfasalazine (4 gm/day). On this regimen the patient's symptoms completely abated, he regained weight, and subsequent sigmoidoscopy and barium enema films were normal. The steroids were gradually tapered and stopped, and the sulfasalazine was maintained at a dosage of 2 gm/day. For the ensuing 7 years he had felt well. He had continued sulfasalazine and had not been seen by a physician for 4 years.

An accountant, he was married with no children and did not use tobacco or alcohol.

At the time of presentation his only complaint was postprandial bloating and flatulence without pain or vomiting. Attempts at lactose exclusion had only a modest effect on the gaseousness. His weight was stable, and he was having two or three semiformed bowel movements per day, with occasional liquid diarrhea after a "rich" meal in a restaurant. His diet was varied, with adequate amounts of protein and complex carbohydrates. He did not take supplemental vitamins. He denied hematemesis, melena, hematochezia, constipation, dyspepsia, fever, skin lesions, arthritis, eye inflammation, aphthous stomatitis, hematuria, kidney stones, and family history of inflammatory bowel disease.

The only significant past medical history was a bleeding duodenal ulcer at age 20 that required surgery to stop the hemorrhage. A vagotomy and an antrectomy with a Billroth II gastrojejunostomy had been performed, and except for twice-daily bowel movements, no symptoms were attributable to the operation.

The physical examination, performed 12 hr after the patient's previous meal, revealed normal vital signs. Other signs were normal except for pale nonicteric conjunctivae; a mildly distended and tympanitic abdomen with normal bowel sounds; a well-healed, midline scar above the umbilicus; and tenderness in the right lower quadrant with the suggestion of a mass. A Hemoccult test was positive.

INITIAL LABORATORY DATA. Hct = 29%; mean corpuscular volume (MCV) = 104 μm^3 with a mixed cell population of micro- and macrocytes; WBC count and erythrocyte sedimentation rate = normal; serum calcium and albumin = low; and electrolytes, liver function, and kidney function = normal. The urinalysis was normal except for large numbers of urate crystals.

A subsequent physical examination performed 1 hr after a meal revealed a distinctly distended tympanitic abdomen and high-pitched bowel sounds. The patient expressed little discomfort at this time.

PHYSIOLOGY

General Considerations

This chapter will describe the mechanisms by which the small intestine handles several important examples of two vital classes of nutrients: minerals (e.g., iron and calcium) and vitamins (e.g., vitamin B_{12} and vitamin A). Space and scope considerations preclude describing the different intestinal absorptive mechanisms for the approximately two dozen minerals and vitamins; the examples described are vital nutrients for health whose gastrointestinal handling is well understood.

Some generalizations are worth noting before considering the specific details of events involved in the assimilation of these four nutrients. Prior to their absorption, these types of nutrients undergo physical and chemical alterations or binding to a transport protein, which either makes the nutrient molecules more soluble in the intestinal fluid or protects the nutrient against degradation by digestive enzymes. These preparatory events are a necessary prelude, without which normal absorption would not occur.

Absorption of these nutrients is by transcellular transport during the postprandial period and involves initial binding to enterocyte receptors for both minerals and vitamin B_{12}. Subsequently, the absorptive process continues inside the enterocyte and may involve synthetic chemical reactions, binding to and release from transport proteins, intracellular diffusion, or active (energy-dependent) transport across the basolateral membrane.

Transcellular transport of iron and calcium is slow and is tightly regulated by negative feedback mechanisms, because maintenance of a relatively fixed store of each mineral in the body is essential. A marked increase or decrease in the concentration of plasma iron or calcium is associated with life-threatening illness.

Iron Absorption

Iron is foremost among the essential minerals required for survival. Iron is a critical element of hemoglobin, which is responsible for the transport of molecular oxygen by red blood cells. Iron is also an essential metal constituent of several redox enzymes, which catalyze the oxidation of organic substrates in cells by molecular oxygen.

Healthy humans maintain a steady level of total body iron during adult life (about 4 gm). This steady amount of iron is maintained by balancing the rate of its absorption against the rate of its loss from the body. Iron is lost at the rate of 1 to 2 mg/day from menstrual bleeding in women and from cell loss, which occurs normally in all people as a result of sloughing of the skin and the epithelial lining of the gastrointestinal tract. If intestinal absorption does not keep up with usual iron losses over a protracted period of time, the end result is an iron deficiency, manifested mostly by anemia that progressively worsens and can be life-threatening.

Iron deficiency is one of the most prevalent and serious nutritional deficiencies worldwide. In the United States, the average adult diet contains about 20 mg of iron per day, which is approximately the recommended daily allowance (RDA) established by the National Academy of Sciences. However, despite ample and inexpensive sources of food containing iron (e.g., hamburgers), along with the extensive consumption of nonprescription multivitamin and mineral supplements that contain iron, iron deficiency remains the most common cause of anemia in the United States. Certain people are more vulnerable to iron deficiency, including substance abusers who do not eat, those on fad diets, anorexics, young women with excessive bleeding during menstruation, and older people with chronic blood loss from gastrointestinal lesions (e.g., ulcers, cancer). The converse problem—chronic absorption of too much iron—can lead to a life-threatening illness known as hemochromatosis. In this disease, excess iron is deposited primarily in the liver and heart and causes fibrotic lesions that impair the normal functions of those vital organs. Fortunately, the fully penetrant, homozygous genetic state of hemochromatosis is uncommon.

Iron is presented to the enterocyte in different forms (Fig. 7–1). Heme is a digestion product of meat, which is absorbed into enterocytes by the process of endocytosis. In the cytosol, ferrous iron (Fe^{++}) is released from heme by heme oxygenase. Dietary ferric iron (Fe^{+++}) is not very soluble in intestinal fluid, so its absorption is very slow. Hydrochloric acid (HCl) in the gastric lumen and dietary ascorbate and citrate in the intestinal lumen reduce Fe^{+++} to Fe^{++}, which is absorbed into the enterocyte much faster. Fe^{++} binds to a receptor in the apical membrane of the enterocyte and is carried into the cytosol by a conformational change in the membrane receptor.

Fe^{++} in the cytosol has two main fates: it can be bound to a storage protein to form the complex known as ferritin, and it can be bound to a transport protein. Ferritin storage of Fe^{++} in the enterocyte is essentially irreversible and represents a loss of absorbed iron to the body. This loss occurs because the half-life of human enterocytes is about 3 days, and enterocytes containing ferritin are sloughed into the lumen, where the iron is lost in the feces. In the other form of intracellular Fe^{++}, the mineral is bound to a transport protein, and Fe^{++} is conveyed to and across the basolateral membrane before being released into the interstitium. The free Fe^{++} is quickly bound to another protein known as transferrin. Transferrin conveys Fe^{++} into the blood and then to the bone marrow, where Fe^{++} is incorporated into hemoglobin in erythrocyte precursor cells.

There are two negative feedback mechanisms that allow the body to decrease the rate of absorption of Fe^{++} from the intestinal lumen when the iron stores in the body are ample and the plasma Fe^{++} concentration is elevated. First, a message is relayed to the enterocyte to reduce the number of Fe^{++} receptors on the apical membrane. This leads to a reduction in the binding of luminal Fe^{++} and, hence, a reduction in the rate of entry of Fe^{++} into the enterocyte. The second negative feedback response to an elevated plasma Fe^{++} concentration is a shift in the production of iron-binding proteins in the upper small intestinal enterocytes. This shift involves an increase in the production of ferritin and a decrease in the production of transport protein. This results in more intracellular storage and less transcellular transport of the Fe^{++} absorbed by the cell from the lumen; therefore, there is less entry of Fe^{++} into the blood.

When the plasma concentration of Fe^{++} is decreased, the negative feedback mechanism operates in the other direction, with an increase in the number of apical mem-

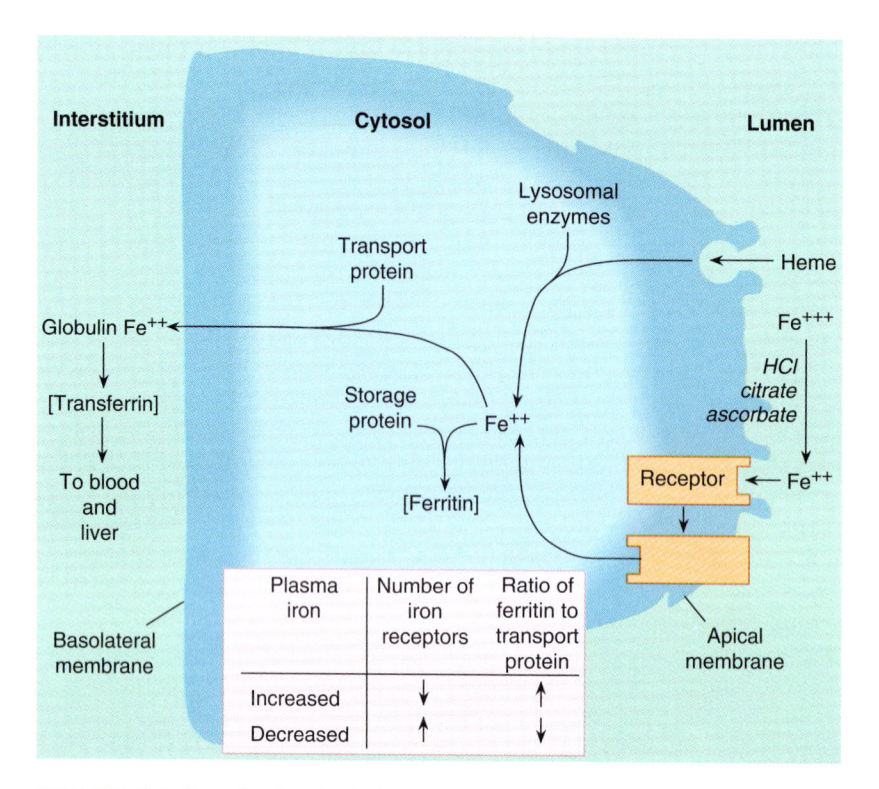

FIGURE 7–1. Iron is absorbed slowly because of complex negative feedback mechanisms. Thus, when plasma [Fe^{++}] levels increase, the number of Fe^{++} receptors diminishes, and the ratio of ferritin (stored Fe^{++} + storage protein in the enterocyte cytosol) to transport protein increases. When plasma [Fe^{++}] levels decrease, opposite effects occur. These changes tend to keep plasma [Fe^{++}] levels fairly constant.

brane receptors and a decrease in the ratio of intracellular production of ferritin versus transport protein. Hence, there is an increase in the rate of uptake of Fe^{++} from the lumen by the enterocyte and an increase in the rate of extrusion of Fe^{++} from the enterocyte into the blood. Although the pathophysiological mechanism of hemochromatosis has not been clearly defined, the disease is probably caused by a breakdown of one or both of the negative feedback mechanisms for iron absorption.

Calcium Absorption

There are ample quantities of calcium (Ca^{++}) in the average American diet, with dairy products and meat being especially rich in this essential nutrient. Ca^{++} is the major component of bone, a critical element in excitable tissues (nerve and muscle), and one of the major second messengers in all cells. Nevertheless, the intestinal absorption of calcium is tightly controlled by a negative feedback mechanism to prevent large swings in the concentration of plasma Ca^{++}. Both hypercalcemia and hypocalcemia are life-threatening abnormalities. The RDA for Ca^{++} is 1 gm.

Before absorption of dietary Ca^{++} can occur, there must be solubilization of this nutrient; this takes place in the acidic gastric juice, where protonation serves to ionize Ca^{++}

(Fig. 7–2). After gastric emptying, Ca^{++} binds to a carrier on the microvillus membrane of the proximal small intestinal enterocyte. After a conformational change of the Ca^{++}-transporter complex, Ca^{++} is relocated to the cytosolic side of the membrane and is released inside the cell. The cytosolic traffic then conveys the Ca^{++} to a Ca^{++}–adenosine triphosphatase (Ca^{++}-ATPase), on the basolateral membrane of the enterocyte, where this Ca^{++} pump actively transports the cation across the cell membrane into the interstitium against a ten-fold higher concentration (extracellular versus intracellular concentrations of Ca^{++}). Ca^{++} enters the blood, thereby raising the plasma concentration and triggering a negative feedback mechanism.

The parathyroid gland responds to the rising plasma Ca^{++} concentration by decreasing the release of parathyroid hormone into the blood. The fall in the delivery of this circulating hormone to the kidney slows a renal chemical reaction that is dependent on the parathyroid hormone—namely, the conversion of vitamin D into 1,25-dihydroxycholecalciferol. The decrease in the delivery of the latter metabolite to the proximal small intestine inhibits the binding of Ca^{++} to the transporters on the apical membrane of upper intestinal enterocytes and reduces the activity of Ca^{++}-ATPase on the basolateral mem-

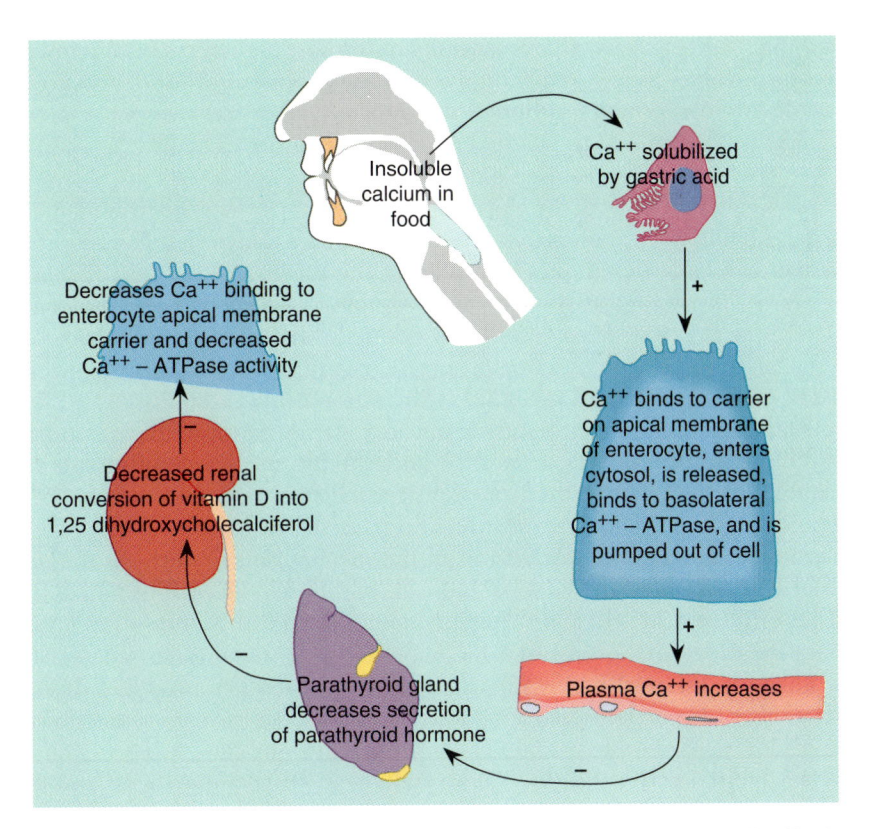

FIGURE 7–2. Absorption of calcium is slow because of a negative feedback mechanism. Accordingly, when plasma [Ca^{++}] levels increase, a message is relayed to the parathyroid gland to decrease secretion of its hormone. Declining plasma parathyroid hormone levels inhibit renal conversion of vitamin D into 1,25-dihydroxycholecalciferol. The diminished synthesis of the latter substance inhibits the binding of intraluminal Ca^{++} to the enterocyte apical membrane carrier and thereby decreases absorption of Ca^{++}. This negative feedback mechanism serves to maintain a steady plasma [Ca^{++}] concentration.

brane. The end result of a rising concentration of Ca^{++} in the plasma is a decrease in the intestinal absorption of Ca^{++}. In the presence of a falling plasma $[Ca^{++}]$ the foregoing process compensates in an opposite manner by increasing the absorption of Ca^{++}.

There are also instances of dysfunction in the absorption of Ca^{++}. Abnormally decreased absorption occurs in three types of disorders: (1) failure to solubilize dietary calcium in the stomach, which occurs in those who chronically consume excessive amounts of antacid medications; (2) loss of microvillus surface area in upper intestinal enterocytes, which occurs in those who suffer malabsorption syndromes such as gluten enteropathy; and (3) saponification of Ca^{++} with excess lipid in the lumen of the duodenum, which occurs in those who suffer malabsorption syndromes in which dietary fat is not digested. Reduced absorption of Ca^{++} over a long period will cause mobilization of the cation from bone, osteomalacia, and spontaneous fractures. Abnormally increased absorption of Ca^{++} leading to hypercalcemia is observed in sarcoid disease.

Vitamins

Vitamins are a sizeable group of chemically and physiologically dissimilar organic compounds that, nevertheless, share several important characteristics. Vitamins are essential for a healthy life, are normally ingested as a component of food, and are required as a regular dietary component, although the daily intake of most vitamins need only be a minute quantity. Vitamins or their immediate precursor forms cannot be synthesized in the body (i.e., they must be consumed either as food or as a pharmaceutical supplement). Vitamins are essential chemicals in vital cell functions such as growth and metabolism. Chronic inaccessibility of a vitamin to the body results in a deficiency disease with a downhill course that can be stopped only by replacing the missing vitamin.

The essential physiological roles of many vitamins, as well as their molecular structure and chemical characteristics, have been defined. Much is also known about the deficiency diseases caused by the absence of specific vitamins. Some better-known examples of this class of essential nutrients include (1) the water-soluble vitamins C and B complex (biotin, cobalamin, folate, niacin, pantothenic acid, pyridoxine, riboflavin, and thiamin); (2) the fat-soluble vitamins A, D, E, and K; and (3) the dietary components that meet some but not all of the criteria listed previously as characteristic of vitamins (e.g., essential amino and fatty acids, choline, inositol, and para-aminobenzoic acid).

As mentioned, a detailed examination of the mechanisms underlying the absorption of more than a dozen different vitamins, most having unique absorptive paths, will not be attempted here. In the case of some vitamins, much is known, whereas for others, information about their intestinal transport is incomplete. Some vitamins and related substances are closely linked to essential bodily processes, and their absence produces dramatic deficiency diseases. For the purposes of this chapter, discussion is restricted to the digestion and absorption of one water-soluble vitamin (cobalamin) and one fat-soluble vitamin (vitamin A). Chapters 5 and 6 describe intestinal absorption of essential amino acids and fatty acids.

COBALAMIN ABSORPTION

Cobalamin, also known as vitamin B_{12}, is a unique biochemical material having an internal organometallic bond between cobalt and carbon. Each of the different forms of cobalamin molecules contains four pyrrole rings linked by methene bridges, a structure reminiscent of that of porphyrin ring compounds. Cobalamin is synthesized only by lower living forms, such as some bacteria. For most humans, the only effective way of obtaining this vitamin is by eating foods high in cobalamin content (e.g., liver, meat, fish, and dairy products). Although certain colonic bacteria synthesize vitamin B_{12}, absorption of cobalamin occurs only in the ileum, which obviates absorption of the endogenously produced vitamin. The total bodily store of cobalamin is 2.5 mg, of which about 70% is located in the liver; the RDA for vitamin B_{12} is 3 μgm. The exclusive ileal absorption and high hepatic concentration of cobalamin suggest that the enterohepatic circulation is an important mechanism for B_{12} preservation in the body. Accordingly, patients who have sustained ileal resection, which interrupts the enterohepatic circulation, develop cobalamin deficiency disease much earlier than do strict vegetarians who consume no B_{12} but whose enterohepatic circulation is intact.

In the human liver, B_{12} is present mainly as adenosyl cobalamin, and the vitamin is located in both mitochondrial and cytosolic compartments of hepatocytes. The two essential metabolic functions of cobalamin are the biosynthesis of succinyl-coenzyme A (succinyl-CoA) and of methionine. Without vitamin B_{12}, neither of these two key metabolites would be generated and over a period of years serious disease would evolve, characterized mainly by megaloblastic anemia and neurological disability.

The different forms of dietary cobalamin have molecular weights of approximately 1000 D and are among the largest dietary molecules regularly absorbed without enzymatic degradation in the gut. A unique and complex mechanism underlies B_{12} absorption and involves several binding proteins of molecular weight 38,000 to 90,000 D. The first step in assimilating cobalamin is to ingest the vitamin in one of its rich food sources. Americans who eat a normal diet and who have no abnormalities of the gastric or ileal mucosae or the pancreas are at essentially no risk of developing cobalamin deficiency.

The process of cobalamin binding to digestive tract proteins begins in the mouth as some B_{12} from chewed food combines with nonintrinsic factor (non-IF) cobalophilins secreted in the saliva (Fig. 7–3). Non-IF cobalophilins are glycoproteins found in saliva, gastric juice, and plasma that bind one cobalamin per molecule. B_{12} bound to non-IF cobalophilins is physiologically inert and cannot be absorbed by the gut in this form. In normal adult plasma, cobalamin is present at concentrations above 200 pg/ml and is mostly bound to cobalophilins. In B_{12} deficiency states the plasma cobalamin concentration falls below 100 pg/ml. After the food is swallowed, cobalamin combines further with salivary and gastric non-IF cobalophilins in the lumen of the stomach.

Human oxyntic cells secrete three products—liquid, protons, and another binding protein—that contribute to preparing vitamin B_{12} for the long trip through the gastrointestinal tract to the absorptive site on the ileal mucosal surface. Gastric juice is composed mainly of water, which dissolves the vitamin and frees it from ingested food. The secreted acid favors continued binding of cobalamin to non-IF cobalophilins in the aqueous solution. However, the major item provided by oxyntic cells for the handling of cobalamin is intrinsic factor (IF), a glycoprotein that binds one cobalamin per IF molecule.

Normal secretagogues of gastric acid secretion stimulate IF release from oxyntic cells. Although free IF in the gastrointestinal lumen is vulnerable to degradation by pepsin and chymotrypsin, once IF binds to cobalamin, the B_{12}-IF complex is resistant to further proteolytic decomposition. The importance of IF to the ultimate absorption of cobalamin is reflected in the following facts: (1) chronic atrophic gastritis in middle-aged adults causes a marked decrease in the number of oxyntic cells of the stomach and can progress to severe atrophy associated with B_{12} deficiency (pernicious anemia), and (2) cobalamin deficiency can be reversed either by injection of synthetic B_{12} or by ingestion of IF (extracted from hog stomachs).

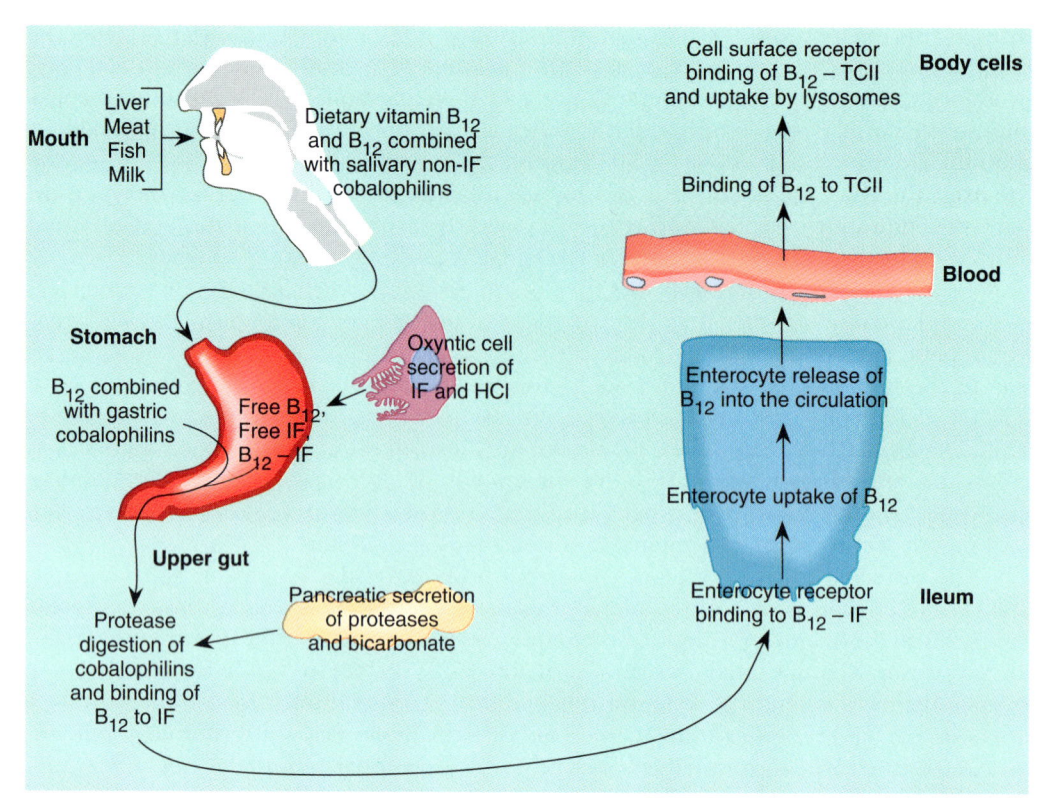

FIGURE 7–3. Gastrointestinal processing of cobalamin consists of multiple sequential steps. It begins with eating foods containing vitamin B_{12} and is followed by the binding of B_{12} to salivary non–intrinsic factor (non-IF) cobalophilins; swallowing of B_{12} and B_{12}-cobalophilin, gastric digestion of food, and liberation of B_{12}; gastric secretion of IF and hydrochloric acid (HCl); gastric emptying of B_{12}, B_{12}–non-IF cobalophilin, and B_{12}-IF; pancreatic secretion of proteases and HCO_3^-; digestion of cobalophilins; B_{12} binding to IF; propulsion of B_{12}-IF to the ileum; enterocyte binding of B_{12}-IF; enterocyte uptake of B_{12} and release of B_{12} into plasma; binding of B_{12} by transcobalamin II (TC II); circulation of B_{12}–TC II to all cells in the body; cell surface receptor binding of B_{12}–TC II; and cellular uptake of B_{12}–TC II into lysosomes.

The human stomach empties its acidic content containing free vitamin B_{12}, B_{12} complexed to either non-IF cobalophilin or IF, and unbound glycoproteins into the duodenum. In the duodenal lumen, the pH is elevated to 6.0 or more, which favors B_{12} binding to IF rather than to non-IF cobalophilin. Inasmuch as pancreatic juice contains proteases, which degrade free non-IF cobalophilins into peptides, as well as high concentrations of HCO_3^-, which elevate luminal pH, nearly all B_{12} binding to IF occurs in the duodenum. Not surprisingly, therefore, patients with pancreatic insufficiency may also exhibit vitamin B_{12} deficiency.

The cobalamin-IF complex is propelled along the gut to the distal 60 cm of the ileum, where specific receptors located on the enterocyte microvilli bind B_{12}-IF. The receptors are essential to the absorption of cobalamin. Conversely, B_{12} bound to non-IF cobalophilins will not bind to the ileal mucosa and will not be absorbed. Some conditions that impair or destroy these receptors and lead to B_{12} deficiency include surgical resection of the ileum, Crohn's disease, bacterial overgrowth, and tropical sprue.

Ileal receptor binding to B_{12}-IF requires Ca^{++} and is optimal at pH 6.6. After the binding step, B_{12}-IF may be transported intact into the enterocyte cytosol, where the complex dissociates and liberates the vitamin inside the cell. Alternatively, the complex may dissociate at the receptor, releasing B_{12} to enter the cell. IF remaining near the receptor will bind any free B_{12} in the ileal lumen for transport into the enterocyte, further cutting cobalamin loss into the feces. The absorption of B_{12}-IF into the cell is an active transport step requiring expenditure of enterocyte energy; it probably uses an unusual mode of transporting the large-molecular-weight complex, such as endocytosis.

Free B_{12} in the enterocyte diffuses into the plasma, where it rapidly binds to transcobalamin II (TC II), a globulin that is synthesized by hepatocytes and enterocytes. As with previous complexing proteins for cobalamin, the molecular binding ratio of TC II to B_{12} is 1:1. Nearly all cells in the body possess a surface receptor that binds the B_{12}–TC II complex, reflecting the essential role of the vitamin in cellular metabolism. After receptor binding, B_{12}–TC II enters the cytosol, where lysosomes take up the complex and degrade TC II. Vitamin B_{12} is freed for intracellular work—namely, participation in the biosynthesis of methionine in the cytosol and succinyl-CoA in the mitochondrion.

VITAMIN A ABSORPTION

Vitamin A_1 is a member of a class of chemically related nutrients known as retinoids. Retinoids are essential for the normal function and structure of epithelial elements, including the eyes, mucous glands, and components of the immune system. Consequently, in vitamin A deficiency, patients suffer loss of night vision and other retinal problems, dermatological lesions, disintegration of mucous glands, and recurrent infections. The first step in incorporating this vitamin is ingesting the nutrient. Vitamin A is plentiful in an ordinary diet, appearing in one form or another in many naturally colorful foods such as egg yolk, corn, tomatoes, butter, yellow beans, liver, green leafy vegetables, mangoes, broccoli, and carrots. The RDA for this vitamin is 5000 IU, and the major storage site in the body is the liver, which normally contains a year's supply of vitamin A.

The most active form of this essential nutrient is vitamin A_1 (all-*trans* retinol) consisting of a beta ionone six-carbon ring to which is attached a nine-carbon side chain containing four double bonds in the *trans* position. The ring is essential for vitamin activity. Vitamin A_1 reaches the intestinal lumen in either free form or as a retinyl ester of palmitic acid. Another related nutrient, beta-carotene, is a provitamin for vitamin A_1. In the lumen, the pancreatic enzyme ester hydrolase dissociates most retinyl ester into vitamin A_1 and the free fatty acid. Another luminal form of the vitamin is retinaldehyde.

The next step in absorbing free vitamin A_1, retinyl ester, and retinaldehyde forms is their emulsification and packaging in micelles, analogous to the digestion of triglycerides as described in Chapter 6. The conjugated bile acids solubilize vitamin A molecules in the aqueous luminal fluid and are critical for forming the micelles, which contain fatty acids, 2-monoglyceride, other lipids, and fat-soluble vitamins, as well as vitamin A molecules. Beta-carotene diffuses directly from the lumen into the cytosol without participating in micelle formation. These early steps and subsequent phases of the absorptive process of vitamin A molecules are depicted in Figure 7–4.

Following the disintegration of the micelles in the unstirred layer and the diffusion of vitamin A_1 and retinaldehyde into the cytosol, these substances undergo re-esterification with long-chain fatty acids (mainly palmitic and stearic acids) and acyl-coenzyme A (acyl-CoA). This resynthesis is facilitated by acyl-CoA–retinol acyltransferase. The newly re-esterified retinyl esters are incorporated into chylomicrons within the cytosol as the vitamin A molecules associate with other dietary lipids that have undergone parallel

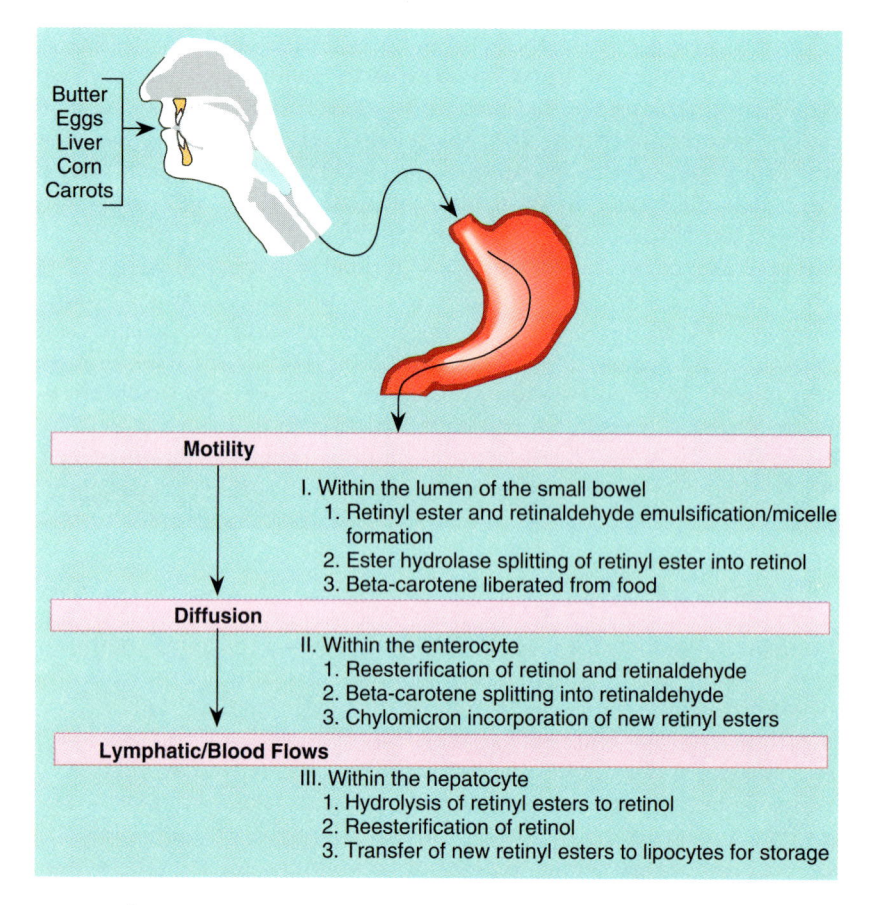

FIGURE 7–4. Gastrointestinal processing of vitamin A molecules. After ingestion and propulsion of food through the upper gastrointestinal tract, vitamin A molecules are solubilized and digested in the gut lumen, diffuse into the enterocyte, undergo intracellular reesterification with fatty acids, and are incorporated into chylomicrons. After circulatory transport in lymphatics and blood vessels, hepatocyte uptake and hydrolysis, and reesterification, the vitamin is stored in hepatic lipocytes.

processes (see Chapter 6). Meantime, beta-carotene is split in the enterocyte cytosol into two molecules of retinaldehyde by the enzyme beta-carotene-15,15-dioxygenase. The retinaldehyde is enzymatically reduced before its reesterification and incorporation into chylomicrons with the other vitamin A molecules.

Chylomicrons are extruded from the enterocyte into the interstitium and migrate into the villus lacteal system. The lymphatics eventually convey the chylomicrons to the systemic venous circulation, which transports vitamin A molecules to the liver. The reesterified retinyl esters are extracted by hepatocytes, hydrolyzed into retinol, reesterified once more with fatty acyl-CoA to form retinyl esters, and transferred within the liver to lipocytes for long-term storage.

Vitamin A deficiency is not a rare pediatric problem in underdeveloped countries, but it is uncommon in the United States. However, hypervitaminosis A has been reported in this country. The serum concentration of vitamin A is fairly constant in humans and is fairly independent of the usual variations in daily intake or amount of vitamin stored in liver lipocytes. However, the availability of over-the-counter vitamin supplements has led to self-medication and overdosage with vitamin A (i.e., chronic intake of more than 10 to 20 times the RDA). Chronic vitamin A toxicity can be detected by a marked elevation in the serum vitamin A concentration and by skin lesions.

CASE REPORT: CONCLUSION

CLINICAL IMPRESSION. Crohn's ileitis in a patient who underwent a partial gastrectomy more than 20 years before presentation with mixed anemia, abdominal distention, and flatulence. His symptoms suggested a chronic distal small bowel stricture and partial obstruction with small bowel bacterial overgrowth caused by Crohn's disease. The potential sources of the mixed anemia were iron deficiency (chronic gastrointestinal blood loss resulting from the Crohn's lesions in the ileum or the partial gastrectomy, poor absorption of dietary iron because of the ulcer operation), folate deficiency (resulting from chronic use of sulfasalazine or bacterial overgrowth), and/or vitamin B_{12} deficiency (resulting from bacterial overgrowth or the ileitis).

RECOMMENDATIONS. Serum ferritin, folate, and vitamin B_{12} were ordered, along with a small bowel series.

The patient was found to have low serum ferritin and low serum B_{12} levels with a normal serum folic acid concentration. The small bowel series demonstrated a high-grade, 20-cm stricture of the terminal ileum with the small bowel dilated proximally to 5 cm in width. Although not confirmed by testing, bacterial overgrowth was assumed in the dilated ileum.

After initiation of therapy with oral ferrous sulfate, vitamin C, and parenteral vitamin B_{12}, the patient's reticulocyte count increased to 10%. A laparotomy was performed, and the strictured ileal segment was removed. Postoperatively the patient's bloating and flatulence disappeared, but he had watery diarrhea. This responded to cholestyramine, and the hematocrit rose to 42%.

CLINICAL OVERVIEW

Mixed anemias may be the presenting problem in some patients with gastrointestinal disease. The most common source of anemia both in the United States and worldwide is iron deficiency, which in turn may be caused by poor diet, menstrual abnormalities, parasites (e.g., hookworm), and gastrointestinal mucosal bleeding. Iron deficiency anemia in young people is usually attributable to one of the first three causes. In elderly people this anemia is more likely the result of a gastrointestinal lesion (e.g., peptic ulcer, gastric cancer, colonic cancer, inflammatory bowel disease). In the case presented in this chapter, the anemia was probably caused by Crohn's disease, in which blood is lost from the inflamed mucosa, coupled with the aftermath of extensive gastric resection. Postsurgical hypochlorhydria interfered with the conversion of Fe^{+++} to Fe^{++}. The patient's reconstructive surgery (Billroth II distal gastrectomy and gastrojejunostomy) also directed ingested food containing iron to bypass the duodenum and most proximal jejunum. These parts of the small bowel are the major normal sites for absorption of iron.

The patient also exhibited a low serum vitamin B_{12} level as well as a decreased serum ferritin concentration; the folate level was normal. The most common cause of a cobalamin deficiency in the United States is pernicious anemia resulting from an atrophic oxyntic cell mass in the stomach. The dearth of oxyntic cells reduces secretion of IF as well as gastric acid. The lack of IF interferes with subsequent cobalamin absorption by the ileal mucosa. Isolated B_{12} deficiency resulting from malnutrition is rare in the United States except in chronic alcoholics and those on long-term macrobiotic (low-protein) diets.

Cobalamin deficiency may result from surgical resection of the terminal 100 cm of the ileum (as treatment for Crohn's disease), which is the locus for mucosal receptors involved in binding the B_{12}-IF complex. Short resections of this region of the ileum are unlikely to precipitate malabsorption of cobalamin. Vitamin B_{12} deficiency may also occur in some patients with pancreatic insufficiency and small bowel bacterial overgrowth (as in obstructive Crohn's disease) in which the bacteria decompose the B_{12}-IF complex.

The Schilling test involves administration of radioactive cobalamin with and without exogenous IF and can distinguish gastric from nongastric causes of vitamin B_{12} deficiency. An abnormally low uptake of B_{12} in the presence of exogenous IF is suggestive of ileal disease. A normal B_{12} uptake with exogenous IF, coupled with low uptake without exogenous IF, suggests pernicious anemia (gastric mucosal disease). An abnormally low B_{12} uptake with and without exogenous IF that is corrected by administration of antibiotics indicates bacterial overgrowth. The Schilling test should not be performed in a patient with an obvious ileal cause of cobalamin deficiency (surgical resection or ileal Crohn's disease). In such a patient, treatment with parenteral vitamin B_{12} satisfies good medical management. Indeed, as a practical matter, once vitamin B_{12} deficiency is established, all patients should be treated with parenteral cobalamin.

CHAPTER EIGHT

Splanchnic Circulation

CASE REPORT: INITIAL INFORMATION

A 58-year-old man was referred to his cardiologist because of episodic abdominal pain and weight loss of 4 months duration. The patient had been in his usual state of health until 4 months previously, when he suffered his first attack of abdominal pain. The pain was knife-like, focused around his umbilicus, occurred toward the end of a large meal, and lasted for 30 min. Initially, the pain recurred every 2 to 3 days; however, during the past month almost every meal was interrupted by the pain. He was afraid to eat and had lost 15 lb. The pain was aggravated by large meals or eating solid food but was not initiated by exercise and was not decreased by antacids, histamine H_2 receptor antagonists, or sublingual nitroglycerine. He had not experienced nausea, vomiting, hematemesis, abdominal bloating, jaundice, constipation, diarrhea, melena, hematochezia, previous stomach operations, or dyspepsia. An upper gastrointestinal series was normal.

His other major medical problem was arteriosclerotic cardiovascular disease, manifested by two myocardial infarctions (the most recent occurring 9 months before presentation); by angina pectoris, treated with verapamil, nitroglycerine as needed, and a single aspirin daily; and by mild congestive cardiac failure, treated with digoxin (0.25 mg/day). He had severe type II hyperlipidemia (cholesterol, 380 mg/dl), treated with diet and lovastatin. He was normotensive and did not smoke cigarettes. His father and paternal grandfather had died of myocardial infarctions before the age of 60.

Physical examination revealed normal vital signs, arcus senilis, xanthelasma, arteriovenous nicking in the fundi, rales in the bases of both lung fields, regular sinus rhythm with a sustained point of maximal impulse, and S_4 gallop without murmurs. The abdominal examination was benign, demonstrating no organomegaly or bruits. A Hemoccult test was positive. There were trace pedal edema and barely palpable dorsalis pedis pulses.

Hemogram, biochemical profile, and thyroid function tests were performed by the referring physician and were normal. A chest radiograph showed a large left ventricle with increased interstitial markings in the lower lung fields. Previous routine radiographs of the abdomen had been normal except for calcifications of the abdominal aorta.

PHYSIOLOGY

General Considerations

The splanchnic circulation is the regional systemic circulation that delivers blood to and from the abdominal viscera, most of which are digestive tract organs. The striking features of the splanchnic circulation are its large size, the diversity of its organs, the complexity of its gross vascular arrangement, and the magnitude of its reservoir function.

The splanchnic circulation is the largest systemic regional circulation of the body. In a 70-kg person, the cardiac output is about 6 L/min, about 30% of which flows through the splanchnic circulation. Its two largest supplying vessels, the celiac and superior mesenteric arteries, are also the two largest branches of the aorta, each with blood flows exceeding those in a renal, common carotid, or iliac artery. The portal vein, which conducts blood from the other splanchnic organs to the liver, has a larger blood flow in the abdomen than does the inferior vena cava at that level of the body. Eventually all of the splanchnic circulation empties into the inferior vena cava from the liver. The appropriate blood flows in the major splanchnic vessels are indicated in Figure 8–1.

The second striking feature of the splanchnic circulation is the heterogeneity of the organs and tissues perfused by this regional vasculature. Splanchnic organs include the liver, gallbladder, stomach, spleen, pancreas, small bowel, colon, and rectum. The functional diversity of these organs makes it difficult to attribute a change in splanchnic arterial blood flow to a change in the function and metabolism of any one organ supplied by that vessel. For example, if celiac artery blood flow increases postprandially, the change could have been caused by increased hepatic metabolism; increased gastric acid secretion;

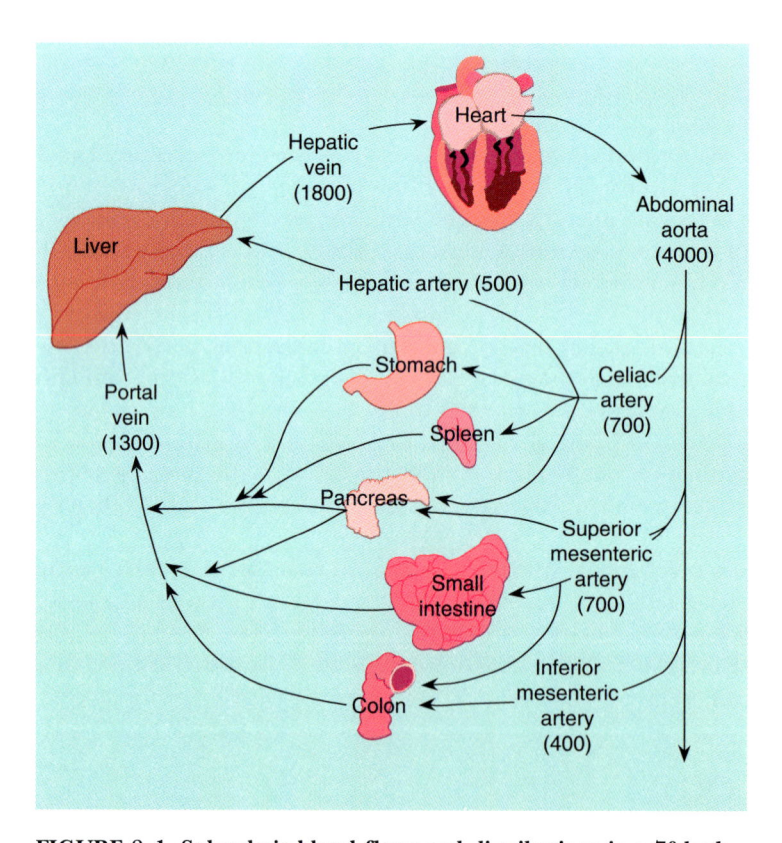

FIGURE 8–1. Splanchnic blood flows and distributions in a 70-kg human. Numbers in parentheses indicate ml/min. The total splanchnic blood flow (1800 ml/min) is equal to (1) the sum of flows in the three inflow vessels (celiac, superior, and inferior mesenteric arteries), (2) the sum of flows in the two inflow vessels to the liver (hepatic artery and portal vein), or (3) the outflow of the hepatic vein.

increased pancreatic enzyme secretion; increased gastroduodenal motility; splenic relaxation; or some combination of these different, organ-specific, functional changes. Furthermore, there is considerable variation in blood flow among the splanchnic organs, among the different tissues in a given organ, and between tissue blood flow in the resting organ and that in the functionally active organ. For example, in the briskly secreting stomach, gastric mucosal blood flow may be increased several times over that in the nonsecreting stomach. Generally, the highest blood flows (per gram of tissue) are observed in the mucosal layers of the hollow gastrointestinal organs. The next highest blood flows (per gram of tissue) are found in the solid organs (pancreas, liver), and the lowest flows occur in the muscular layers of the hollow organs.

The arrangement of blood vessels in the splanchnic circulation is complicated, because the venous drainage of most splanchnic organs flows to the liver rather than directly into the inferior vena cava. Furthermore, the liver receives blood flow from both arterial and venous sources. Consequently, total hepatic blood flow or hepatic vein blood flow is equal to total splanchnic blood flow, and portal venous blood flow is equal to total splanchnic blood flow minus hepatic artery blood flow. These relationships are apparent in Figure 8–1.

The reservoir function of the splanchnic veins and venules is massive compared with that of any other systemic regional circulation. In a 70-kg adult, the total blood volume is about 6 L, one third of which is located in the splanchnic circulation. With general stimuli, such as heavy exercise, that mobilize blood into the venous return to the heart and lungs, nearly 2 L of blood is recruited centrally from the body's many peripheral circulations. Of this mobilized volume, two thirds will have been squeezed out of the venules of the liver, spleen, and gut (Fig. 8–2).

FIGURE 8–2. Total blood volume and mobilized blood volume in splanchnic organs compared with the rest of the body. Although the liver, spleen, and gut compose less than a tenth of body weight, they contain one third of the total blood volume and two thirds of the blood that can be mobilized centrally in response to exercise or other stresses.

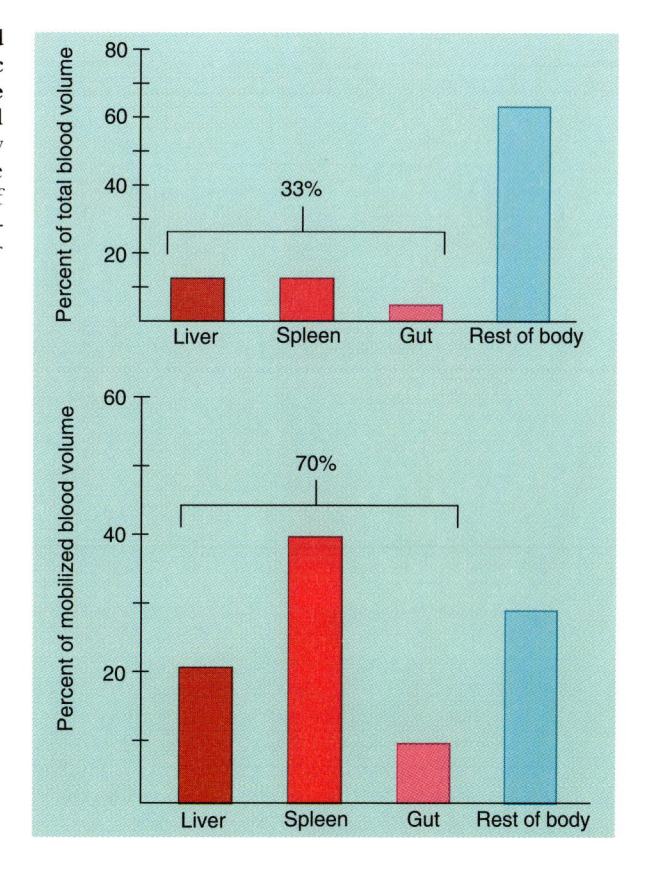

Splanchnic Hemodynamics

In the splanchnic circulation, as in other peripheral vascular beds, the hemodynamic characteristics can be described using three measurable parameters: blood flow, blood pressure, and vascular resistance. These three parameters are related as follows:

$$\text{Vascular resistance} = \frac{\text{Blood pressure}}{\text{Blood Flow}} = \text{mm Hg/ml per min}$$

At a mean arterial pressure of 100 mm Hg and mean superior mesenteric artery blood flow of 700 ml/min, vascular resistance in this artery would be 0.14 mm Hg/ml per min.

Vascular resistance is the force that has to be overcome by blood pressure to permit flow through a blood vessel. Vascular resistance reflects the tension developed by the smooth muscle walls of the blood vessel. Most of the resistance to blood flow occurs in the microscopic arteries (Fig. 8–3). In these high-resistance vessels, the smooth muscle wall is relatively thicker, compared with the vascular lumen, than in visible arteries, capillaries, or veins. Therefore, the major site of blood flow regulation in the circulation of an organ, such as the gut, resides in these high-resistance arterioles. Accordingly, if a drug is to change mesenteric blood flow, the agent has to act mainly on the tension of the arterioles. For example, systemic administration of norepinephrine at some dose will double vascular resistance in the superior mesenteric artery and increase arterial pressure by 50%. The result, using the equation given earlier, would be a 23% reduction in blood flow from 700 to 536 ml/min.

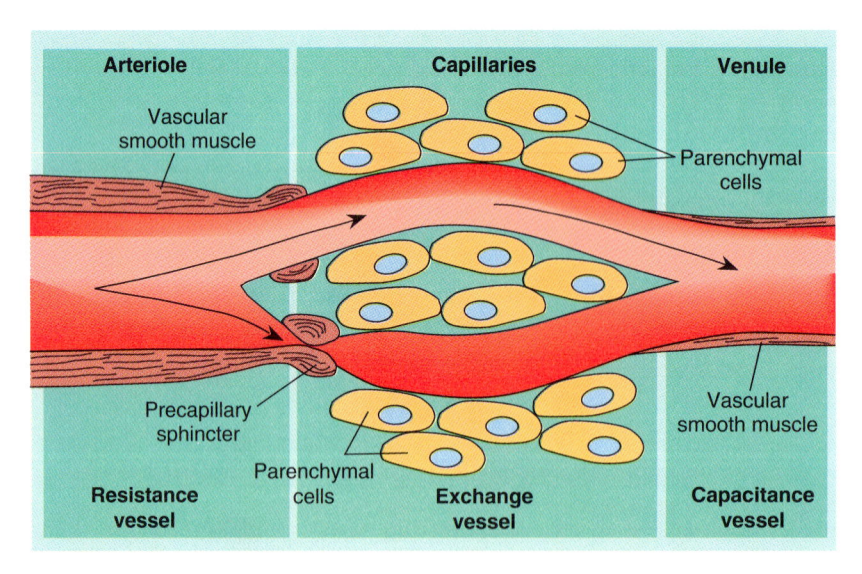

FIGURE 8–3. Structures of the mesenteric microcirculation and their functions. Arterioles are microscopic arteries (<50-μm diameter) with relatively thick, vascular, smooth muscle walls. They generate most of the resistance to blood flow in the entire circulation and thus are the major sites for control of blood flow. Capillaries have thin nonmuscular walls that provide a medium for exchange of oxygen, solutes, and fluids between blood and parenchymal cells. Blood flow through capillaries is controlled by precapillary sphincters, and not all capillaries are open at once. The thin muscular walls of venules allow for capacitance of large volumes of blood.

Vasoconstriction and vasodilation are terms used to describe the effects of physiological, pharmacological, or pathological influences on vascular resistance. An intervention that increases vascular resistance is said to be a vasoconstrictor event, (e.g., sympathetic nerve stimulation, norepinephrine injection [as in the earlier example] or essential hypertension). Vasoconstriction occurs when only the arterial pressure increases, only the blood flow decreases, or both changes take place. There are multiple naturally occurring splanchnic vasoconstrictor agents in the body, such as norepinephrine, angiotensin II, vasopressin, Ca^{++}, endothelins, and prostaglandin $F_{2\alpha}$. The major cellular mechanism responsible for splanchnic vasoconstriction involves the accumulation of Ca^{++} inside the vascular myocyte (Fig. 8–4).

Vasodilation occurs when vascular resistance decreases. Vasodilation may result from relaxation of arteriolar smooth muscle in response to physiological, pharmacological, or pathological influences such as an increase in tissue metabolism, an antihypertensive therapy, or a severe anemia. Vasodilation may be caused by an increase in blood flow only, a decrease in arterial pressure only, or both. There are many naturally occurring vasodilator agents in the splanchnic circulation, such as catecholamines acting on beta$_2$-adrenergic receptors, acetylcholine, adenosine, neuropeptide transmitters, nitric oxide (NO), bradykinin, prostacyclin, and histamine. Two major mechanisms responsible for vasodilation involve the accumulation of either cyclic AMP or cyclic GMP in vascular smooth muscle cells (Fig. 8–5).

Control of Splanchnic Blood Flow

Blood flow in the splanchnic circulation is determined by several major regulatory factors, including general cardiovascular hemodynamics, autonomic nerves, circulating vasoactive materials, local tissue metabolism, and local vascular properties (Fig. 8–6). Each of these factors is sufficiently influential under normal circumstances to justify additional consideration.

General cardiovascular hemodynamics refers to circulatory forces and their relationships, which are represented by cardiac output, systemic arterial blood pressure, blood volume, viscosity of circulating blood, and total peripheral resistance. A major deviation in one or more of these general hemodynamic parameters will evoke a significant change in splanchnic blood flow. For example, after acute hemorrhage of 2 L of blood in an adult

FIGURE 8–4. Norepinephrine contracts the arteriole and increases its intracellular [Ca^{++}]. An intracellular Ca^{++} probe (FURA-2) that binds Ca^{++} and emits detectable biofluorescence was used to determine cytosolic [Ca^{++}] before and after addition of norepinephrine. The excised mesenteric arterial branch had a resting diameter of 60 μm (*left*) and emitted biofluorescent colors indicating an intracellular [Ca^{++}] of 150 nM. Addition of norepinephrine to the bathing medium at a concentration of 30 nM evoked a 50% decrease in vessel diameter and a fourfold increase in cytosolic [Ca^{++}], as indicated by the change in biofluorescent colors. (Courtesy of Omar D. Hottenstein, Ph.D.)

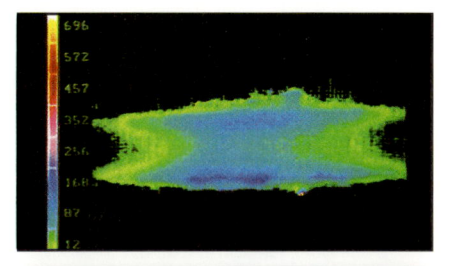

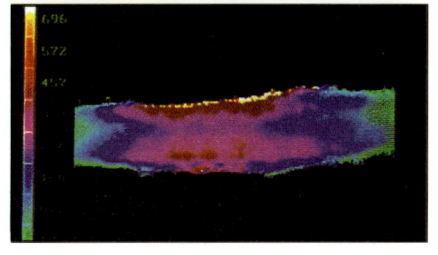

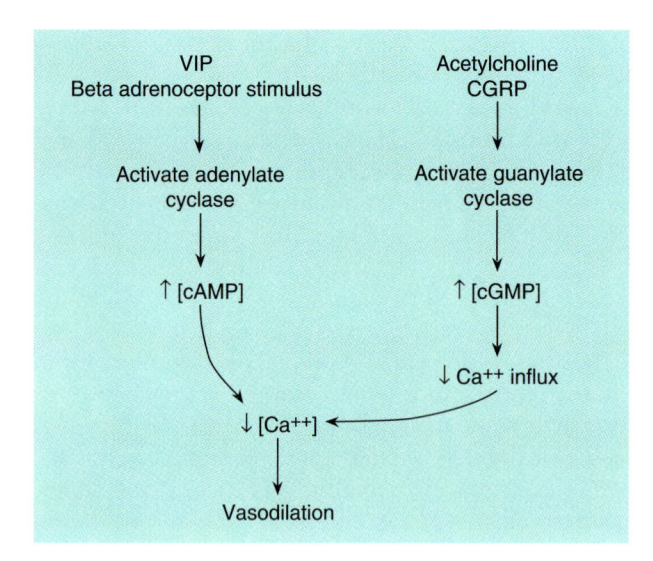

FIGURE 8–5. Increasing vascular muscle intracellular cyclic nucleotide concentrations leads to vasodilation. Certain vasodilator interventions, such as release of vasoactive intestinal peptide (VIP) or stimulation of beta-adrenergic receptors, activate adenylate cyclase conversion of adenosine triphosphate (ATP) into cyclic adenosine monophosphate (cAMP) inside the muscle cell. Other vasodilator interventions, such as release of acetylcholine or calcitonin gene–related peptide (CGRP), activate guanylate cyclase conversion of guanosine triphosphate (GTP) into cGMP within the muscle cell. Buildup of cyclic nucleotide concentrations leads to a lowering of cytosolic [Ca^{++}] and relaxation of the muscle cell.

male, the blood volume shrinks, the venous return to the heart declines abruptly, and the cardiac output is reduced dramatically (Fig. 8–7). As a result, systemic arterial blood pressure decreases, and total peripheral resistance increases. Not surprisingly, splanchnic blood flow is markedly reduced, and splanchnic vascular resistance is increased, reflecting the hypotension, ischemia, and vasoconstriction in the gastrointestinal and hepatic circulations.

Several components of the autonomic nervous system can influence the splanchnic circulation. The extrinsic nerves include sympathetic, parasympathetic, and primary sensory fibers. The intrinsic nerves are branches of the enteric nervous system located in the

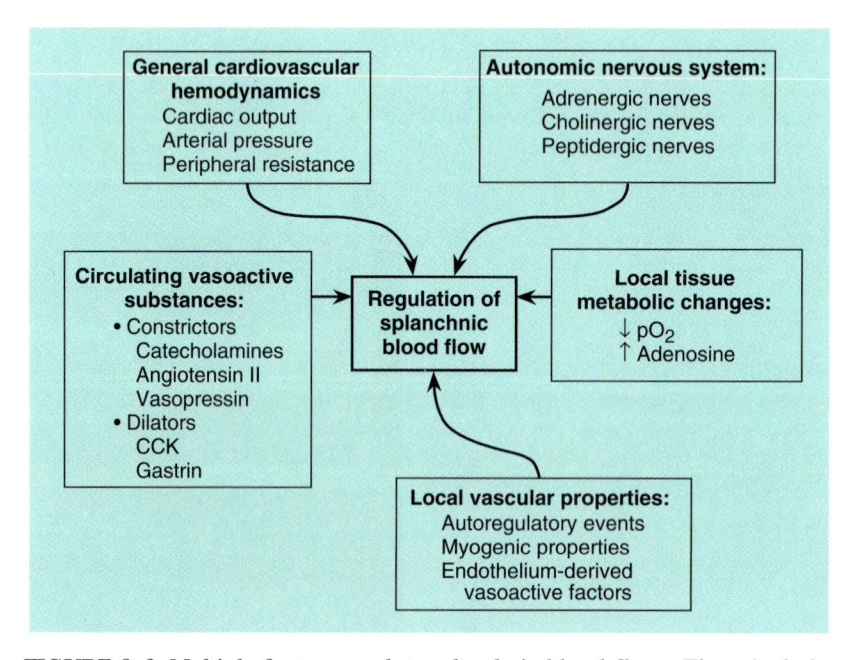

FIGURE 8–6. Multiple factors regulate splanchnic blood flows. These include general cardiovascular hemodynamics, autonomic nerves, circulating vasoactive substances, tissue metabolism, and intrinsic vascular properties.

```
2 liter blood loss
        ↘
    Reduced blood volume
            ↘
        Decreased venous return
                ↘
            Heart
                ↘
            Decreased cardiac output
                    ↘
                Reduced arterial pressure
                        ↘
                    Increased total
                    peripheral resistance
                            ↘
                        Decreased splanchnic
                        blood flows
```

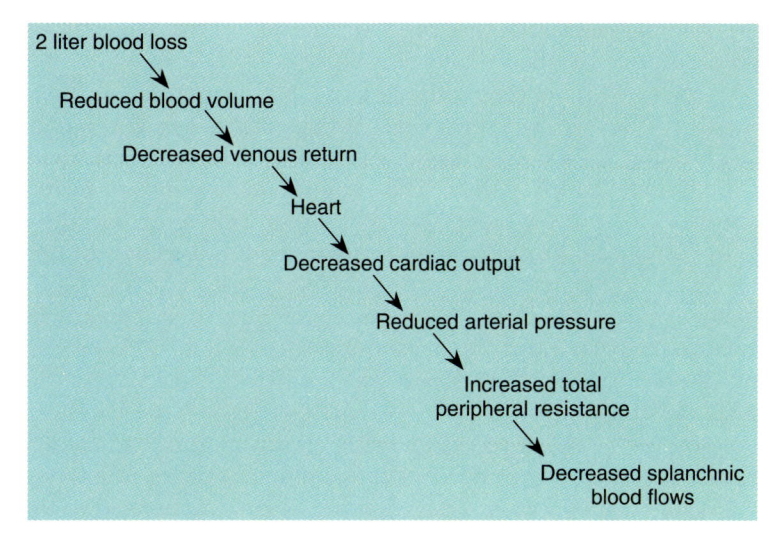

FIGURE 8–7. Severe hemorrhage adversely affects general cardiovascular hemodynamics on which splanchnic blood flow depends. Blood loss from anywhere in the body will reduce blood flow from the heart to the splanchnic organs, diminish the driving force of arterial pressure, and increase the resistance to blood flow in the peripheral vasculature (e.g., splanchnic vessels).

myenteric and submucosal plexuses. Many different neurotransmitter agents are released by the autonomic nerves (Fig. 8–8).

Sympathetic postganglionic motor nerves arise in the prevertebral ganglia (celiac, superior mesenteric, inferior mesenteric, and hypogastric) and project into the viscera in the perivascular splanchnic nerve trunks. At the nerve terminus, norepinephrine is re-

Autonomic divisions with vasoactive neurotransmitters	Vasoconstrictor transmitters	Vasodilator transmitters
Sympathetic nerves	Catecholamines acting on alpha-2 receptors	Catecholamines acting on beta-2 receptors
Parasympathetic nerves		Acetylcholine VIP
Primary sensory nerves	Neuropeptide Y	CGRP Substance P Nitric oxide
Enteric nerves		Acetylcholine VIP

FIGURE 8–8. Splanchnic vessels are constricted or dilated by different types of autonomic nerves that release vasoactive neurotransmitters. The four autonomic divisions that regulate splanchnic blood flow include sympathetic, parasympathetic, primary afferent, and intrinsic enteric nerves. Their vasoactive neurotransmitters include catecholamines, acetylcholine, several neuropeptides, and nitric oxide (NO).

leased into the synaptic cleft adjoining the vascular smooth muscle cell membrane. Alpha$_2$-adrenergic receptors on the cell surface bind norepinephrine and elicit acute contraction of the muscle cell via an increased flux of Ca^{++} from the extracellular compartment and release of Ca^{++} from intracellular stores (Fig. 8–9). Norepinephrine is also bound to beta$_2$-adrenergic receptors on the vascular muscle cell surface, which leads to relaxation of the muscle cell over time. Thus, the initial response to norepinephrine is an abrupt decrease in mesenteric blood flow, which gradually returns to the control value that existed before norepinephrine, despite continued administration of norepinephrine (Fig. 8–10).

Parasympathetic fibers are distributed to the splanchnic viscera mainly from branches of the vagus nerves. Acetylcholine, the major transmitter, is a vasodilator substance in the splanchnic circulation. Acetylcholine is also released by intrinsic nerves in the enteric plexuses (see Fig. 8–8).

Primary sensory nerves have receptors in the gastrointestinal mucosae that are activated by a variety of stimuli such as nutrients in the lumen, reduced blood flow, and adrenergic nerve stimulation. These sensory nerves project from the mucosa to the spinal cord via dorsal root ganglia; they also project to the prevertebral sympathetic ganglia. Their axons travel mainly in the perivascular nerve trunks, and their transmitters are neuropeptides such as calcitonin gene–related peptide (CGRP), substance P, and VIP. These neurotransmitters are also potent vasodilator agents in the splanchnic circulation. Hence, they are referred to as nonadrenergic, noncholinergic (NANC) vasodilator nerves. Activation

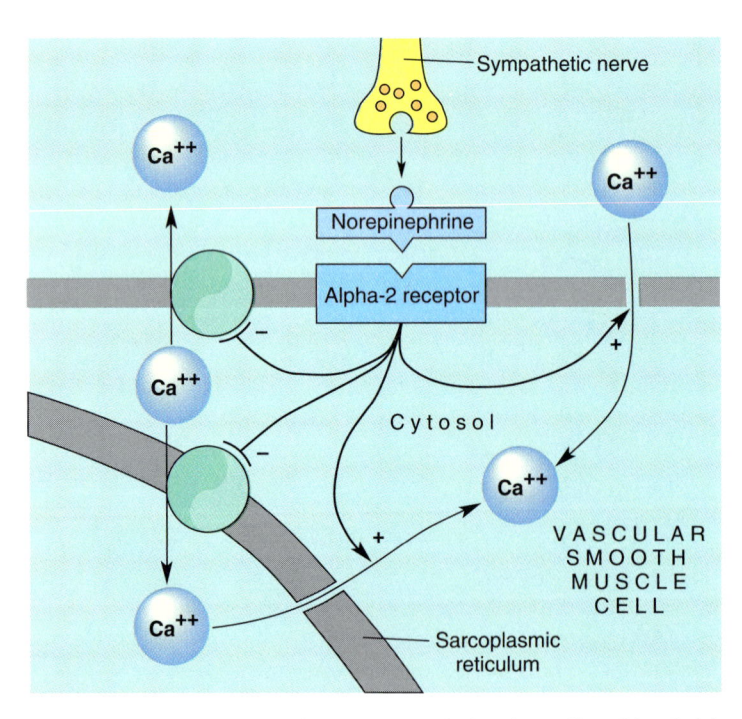

FIGURE 8–9. Norepinephrine vasoconstriction is mediated by Ca^{++} buildup in the cytosol of the vascular muscle cell. The intracellular [Ca^{++}] is increased by enhancing (+) the slow inward diffusion of Ca^{++} from the extracellular space, by prompting (+) Ca^{++} release from sarcoplasmic reticulum, and by inhibiting (−) active transport of Ca^{++} out of the cytosol.

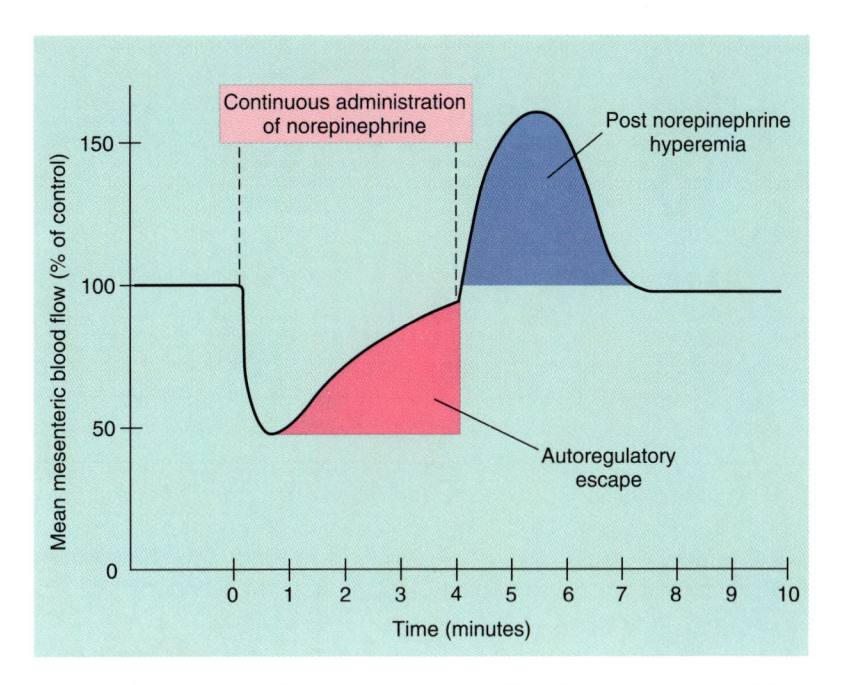

FIGURE 8–10. Autoregulatory events surrounding the mesenteric arterial response to norepinephrine. Initially, norepinephrine constricts intestinal resistance vessels and decreases blood flow. Then, despite continuous administration of norepinephrine, blood flow recovers toward the prenorepinephrine control value. This partial recovery is termed "autoregulatory escape." After cessation of norepinephrine administration, there is a transient overshoot in blood flow to a level well above the control value. This overshoot is termed "post norepinephrine hyperemia." These autoregulatory events are dilator responses that depend on several mediators such as beta-adrenergic receptors, primary afferent neuropeptides, adenosine release, and NO.

of NANC nerves elicits intestinal vasodilation by two pathways (Fig. 8–11). First, there is a long reflex to the spinal cord and superior mesenteric ganglion that inhibits sympathetic nervous release of norepinephrine. There is also a short reflex to the arterioles that releases NANC vasodilator peptides near the arteriolar wall. The cellular mechanisms whereby NANC neuropeptides elicit vasodilation are shown in Figure 8–5.

Circulating vasoactive substances may alter blood flow to splanchnic organs directly or indirectly. Catecholamines, angiotensin II, and vasopressin act directly on the vascular wall (smooth muscle or endothelium) to elicit constrictor responses and reduce splanchnic blood flow and blood volume. However, the conditions that prompt release of these blood-borne, direct vasoconstrictor agents are unusual (e.g., severe exercise, oligemic shock, congestive cardiac failure). More usual circulating materials that increase mesenteric blood flow and that are released regularly at mealtimes include endocrine peptides such as gastrin, cholecystokinin (CCK), and secretin. These hormones stimulate postprandial events such as exocrine secretion and gastrointestinal motility, thereby increasing the metabolism of parenchymal cells.

With augmented parenchymal metabolism, there is postprandial vasodilation and increase in blood flow to the stomach, pancreas, gut, and liver (Fig. 8–12). The mediation of metabolically induced vasodilation involves changes in the chemical environment near the vascular smooth muscle of the precapillary sphincters (see Fig. 8–3). The mediators

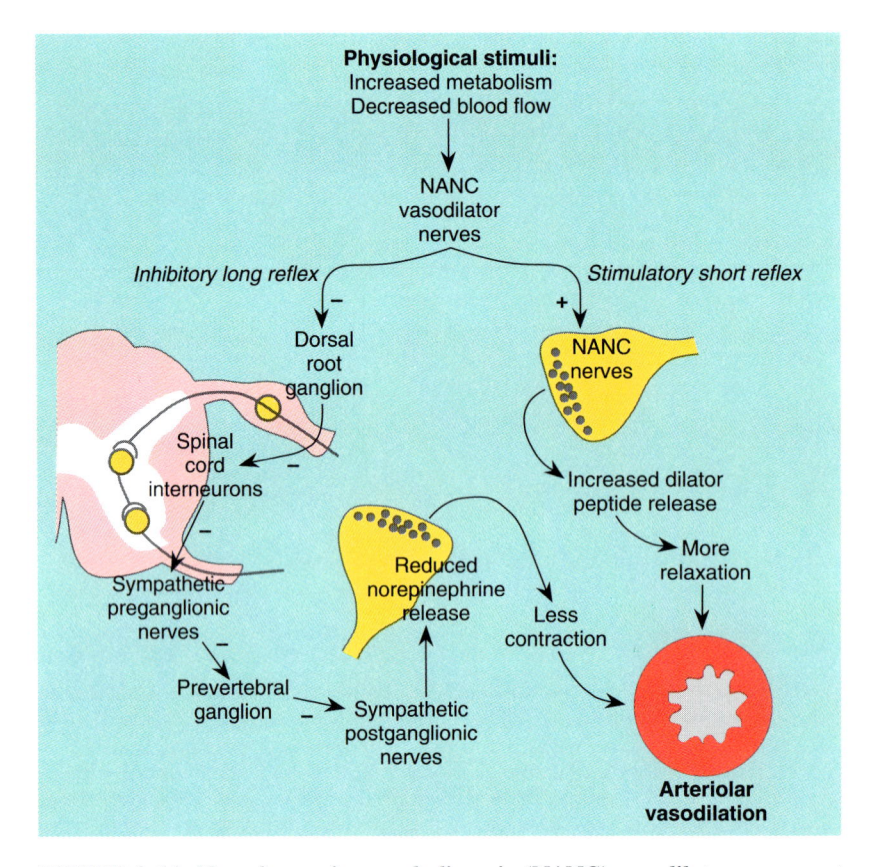

FIGURE 8–11. Nonadrenergic, noncholinergic (NANC) vasodilator nerves act via two reflexes. The physiological stimuli are either enhanced splanchnic metabolism (as during mealtime) or diminished splanchnic blood flow (as during exercise). The long reflex via the spinal cord inhibits (−) sympathetic neural release of norepinephrine, thereby attenuating arteriolar constriction. The short reflex involves direct NANC neuropeptide release, which stimulates (+) arteriolar vasodilation.

of metabolic relaxation of blood vessels include low pO_2 and adenosine release. Relaxation of precapillary muscle increases the density of perfused capillaries and thereby increases the availability of oxygen and blood-borne nutrients to support the higher cellular metabolism.

The intrinsic properties of splanchnic blood vessels also influence blood flow in this circulation. Three types of endogenous circulatory mechanisms have been described in splanchnic vessels: autoregulatory events, myogenic properties, and endothelial phenomena.

Autoregulation is the ability of the circulation of an organ to vasodilate in response to increased metabolism or decreased blood flow. Autoregulation depends on local mechanisms (i.e., it is independent of extrinsic innervation or circulating vasoactive substances). Examples of intestinal autoregulatory events include postprandial hyperemia, which is an increase in mesenteric blood flow in response to the intraluminal instillation of micellar lipid and saline, and escape from continuous vasoconstrictor input with sympathetic nerve stimulation or administration of norepinephrine. Both of these autoregulatory phenomena depend on local intestinal mechanisms such as intrinsic afferent nerves, endothelial factors, and adenosine release.

FIGURE 8–12. The enhanced postprandial metabolism increases capillary blood flow and the availability of oxygen and nutrients. As oxygen is consumed and dilator metabolites, such as adenosine, are released, precapillary sphincters relax, thereby opening more capillaries to the flow of blood. In this way the blood and the actively metabolizing cells can exchange more oxygen and nutrients.

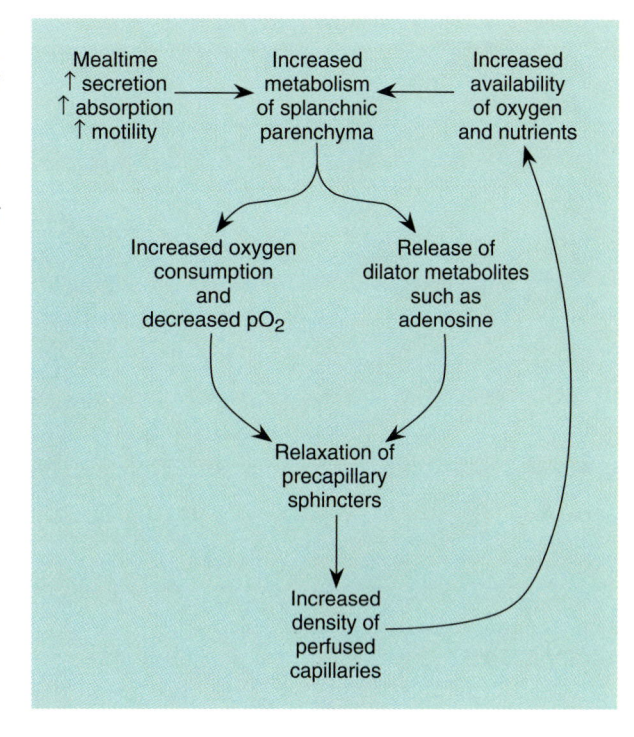

Myogenic properties of arterioles involve active relaxation of the vascular wall in response to a decrease in blood pressure that otherwise would have caused a decreased blood flow. Conversely, the arterioles contract when blood pressure is elevated, thereby offsetting an otherwise unchecked increase in blood flow. Such responses serve to maintain blood flow at an optimal value for the involved organ. Myogenic properties depend on the intrinsic stretch of vascular muscle and endothelial reactions to the increased velocity of flowing blood.

The endothelium of mesenteric microcirculatory vessels synthesizes and releases several vasodilator agents such as prostacyclin, bradykinin, and NO. NO, a relaxing factor, seems to be the necessary intermediate for several other vasodilator mediators such as CGRP, bradykinin, and acetylcholine (Fig. 8–13). NO is synthesized in the endothelial cell and diffuses into the adjacent smooth muscle cell, where it reduces intracellular $[Ca^{++}]$, thereby relaxing the vascular muscle.

The foregoing array of factors and mediators that contribute to vasodilation in the gut are depicted in Figure 8–14. The complexity of local regulation of mesenteric vasodilation is attributable to several cell types that generate numerous vasoactive agents, many of which can stimulate release of other vasodilator materials.

Mesenteric Circulation

The small and large bowel together constitute 6% of total body weight and contain 7% of total body blood volume. However, when blood is mobilized from all peripheral circulations in response to stress, such as heavy exercise, the intestines contribute 10% of all the mobilized blood. In a 70-kg adult, blood flow to the gut is about 1 L/min, which is 60% of the total splanchnic blood flow. The mesenteric circulation is distributed nearly equally between the small intestine and the colon/rectum.

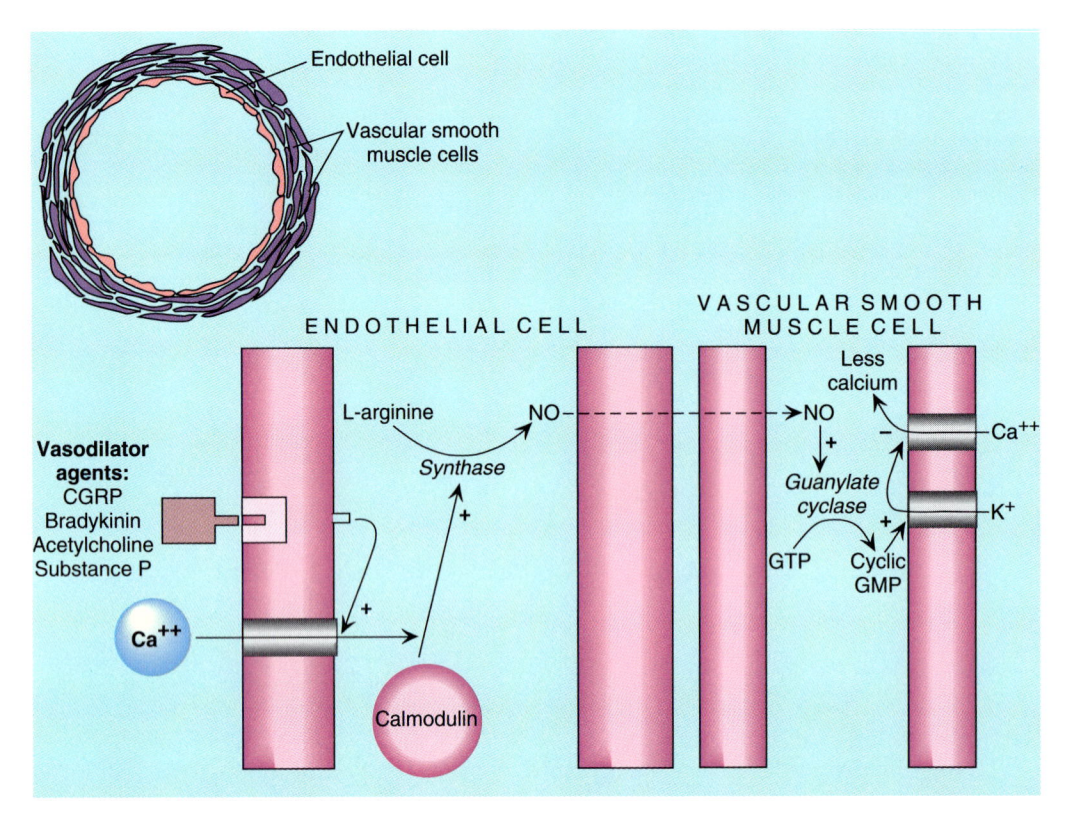

FIGURE 8–13. Endothelial NO is a key intermediary for the action of several neurovasodilator agents. When one of these agents binds to endothelial cell surface receptors, there is stimulation (+) of Ca^{++} influx, and Ca^{++} binds to an intracellular protein, calmodulin. The Ca^{++}-calmodulin complex activates synthesis of NO in the endothelial cytosol. NO diffuses into nearby vascular muscle cells, where it stimulates production of cyclic GMP. The nucleotide opens K^+ channels, which hyperpolarize the muscle cell membrane, decrease (−) Ca^{++} influx, relax the cell, and cause vasodilation.

The major recurring physiological event in the mesenteric circulation is mealtime. Postprandially, intestinal blood flow increases from resting values and reaches peak values (+25% to +100% of resting flow) at 30 to 90 min after ingestion of food. This increase in mesenteric blood flow, prompted by eating and the propulsion of nutrients into the small intestinal lumen, is termed "postprandial hyperemia." Small degrees of postprandial hyperemia can be elicited by infusing isosmotic saline into the jejunal lumen. However, the full expression of this autoregulatory increase in mesenteric blood flow occurs when nutrients are propelled into the lumen, especially micellar lipid (>20 mmol/L oleate dissolved in a solution containing 10% bile and 90% isosmotic saline). The principal mechanisms underlying postprandial hyperemia are local neural, metabolic, and endocrine factors—namely, NANC neuropeptides, cholinergic transmitters, decreased pO_2, and release of adenosine, CCK, and bradykinin.

Accompanying the enhanced blood flow of postprandial hyperemia is an increase in oxygen consumption, which reflects an increase in metabolic work associated with mucosal digestion and absorption of nutrients. Most of the augmented blood flow is delivered to the mucosa. There is a positive correlation among mucosal active cotransport of glucose and sodium, oxygen consumption, and blood flow. The mechanism linking these

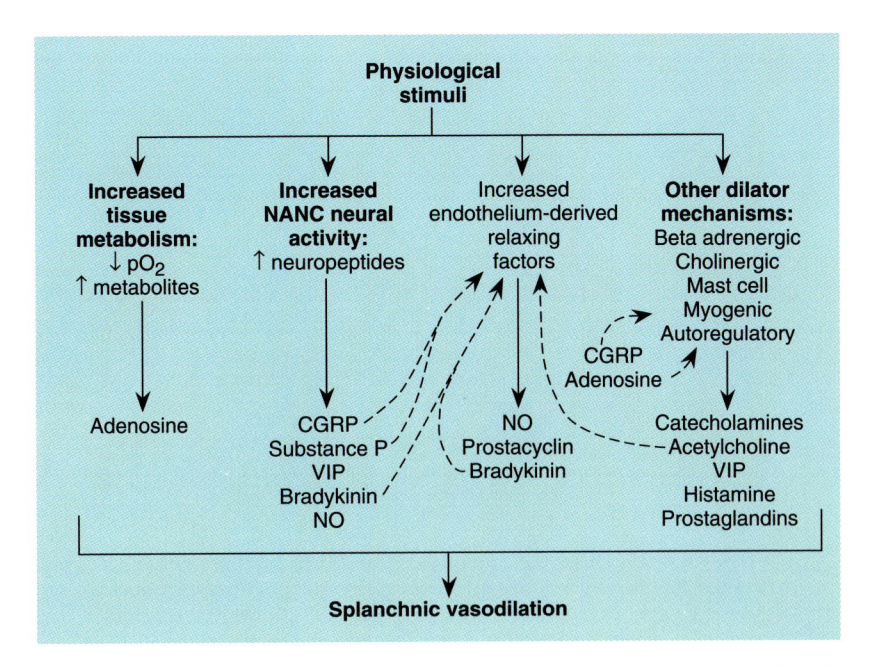

```
                    Physiological
                      stimuli
     ┌──────────┬──────────┬──────────┬──────────┐
     ▼          ▼          ▼                     ▼
Increased   Increased   Increased          Other dilator
  tissue   NANC neural endothelium-derived mechanisms:
metabolism:  activity:    relaxing         Beta adrenergic
  ↓ pO₂    ↑ neuropeptides factors          Cholinergic
↑ metabolites                                  Mast cell
                                               Myogenic
                                             Autoregulatory
                                    CGRP
                                   Adenosine
     ▼          ▼          ▼                     ▼
 Adenosine    CGRP        NO              Catecholamines
            Substance P  Prostacyclin     -- Acetylcholine
              VIP        Bradykinin            VIP
            Bradykinin                       Histamine
              NO                           Prostaglandins
     └──────────┴──────────┬──────────┴──────────┘
                           ▼
                 Splanchnic vasodilation
```

FIGURE 8–14. Numerous vasodilator mechanisms and mediators act directly and through one another to increase splanchnic blood flow. Vasodilation of splanchnic organs involves metabolic, neural, endothelial, immunological, and muscle cell processes and acts through the release of many specific dilator mediators. These mediators can relax vascular muscle directly or can amplify their vasodilator effects by invoking the release of other mediators (*dashed arrows*).

functional parameters is a mucosal microcirculatory change—namely, the relaxation of smooth muscle in the precapillary sphincters (see Fig. 8–3). This muscle relaxation is presumably mediated by local metabolic factors such as a lower pO_2 (see Fig. 8–12). The result is an opening of more mucosal capillaries for perfusion with blood containing oxygen and nutrients to support the metabolically active absorbing enterocytes.

Increases in intestinal blood flow and oxygen uptake differ depending on the stimulus involved. With active cotransport of glucose and Na^+, there is a small increase in blood flow and a comparable increase in oxygen extraction (i.e., the arteriovenous oxygen concentration difference across the gut). Hence, intestinal oxygen consumption (i.e., blood flow × the arteriovenous oxygen difference) increases more proportionately than does blood flow. By contrast, certain vasodilator agents (e.g., adenosine) increase blood flow proportionately more than they increase oxygen consumption. These differences are shown in Figure 8–15 and reflect various microcirculatory sites being affected by the foregoing stimuli. Accordingly, when mucosal pO_2 decreases and relaxes precapillary sphincters, thereby opening more capillaries to the flow of blood, the arteriovenous oxygen difference increases, and oxygen consumption increases proportionately more than does blood flow. With a vasodilator agent such as adenosine, the major microcirculatory muscles being relaxed are the myocytes surrounding the arterioles, which are the prime regulators of blood flow to the gut. In this situation, blood flow increases proportionately more than does oxygen uptake, because the arteriovenous oxygen difference actually decreases.

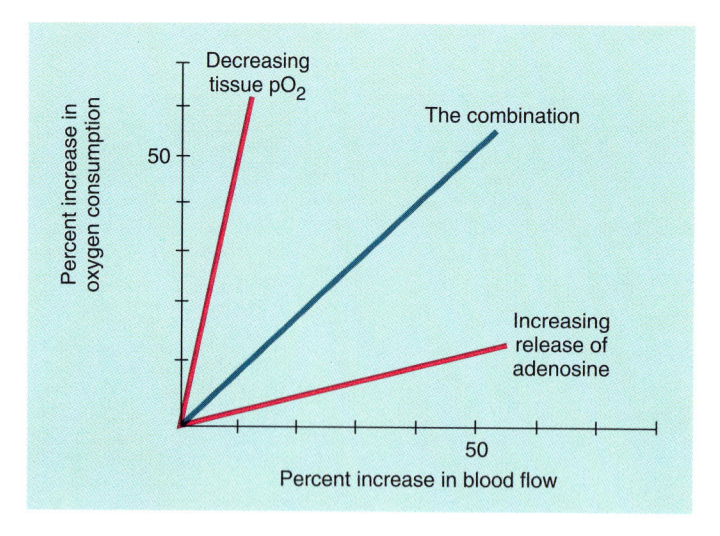

FIGURE 8–15. Different metabolic stimuli can increase either intestinal blood flow or oxygen consumption proportionately more. As tissue pO_2 declines during active gut metabolism, the arteriovenous oxygen concentration difference across the gut will increase along with blood flow. Oxygen consumption is the product of the arteriovenous oxygen difference and blood flow and will therefore increase faster than the increase in blood flow. Adenosine release affects mainly resistance vessels and increases blood flow, while the arteriovenous oxygen difference decreases. Therefore, the increase in blood flow is proportionately greater than the increase in oxygen consumption.

Hepatic Circulation

The liver is the largest solid splanchnic organ, constituting about 3% of total body weight. Inasmuch as the entire splanchnic circulation (30% of cardiac output) perfuses the liver via the portal vein and hepatic artery, resting blood flow through the liver is high, amounting to about 100 ml/min per 100 gm hepatic tissue. Nearly three fourths of liver blood flow is supplied by the portal vein (see Fig. 8–1). Mean hepatic artery and portal vein blood pressures are approximately 100 mm Hg and 10 mm Hg, respectively.

Changes in vascular resistance within the liver influence hepatic arterial perfusion reciprocally (e.g., increased intrahepatic resistance causes decreased hepatic artery blood flow). Although increased intrahepatic resistance raises the portal venous pressure, the control of portal vein blood flow is determined mainly by changing arterial resistances in the other splanchnic organs from which blood drains into the portal circulation. Thus, a decrease in mesenteric vascular resistance will elicit an increase in blood flow through the gut and into the mesenteric branches of the portal vein. Portal vein blood flow will increase. The major sources of blood flowing into the portal vein are the small and large bowel (60%), stomach (20%), spleen (10%), and pancreas (10%). From the foregoing considerations, the two vessels supplying blood to the liver differ hemodynamically. For example, the hepatic artery has a high vascular resistance (0.20 mm Hg/ml per min), whereas the portal vein has a much lower resistance (0.01 mm Hg/ml per min).

Hepatic arterial blood flow is not affected much by changes in hepatic metabolism. However, hepatic arterial blood flow is influenced reciprocally by changes in portal vein blood flow. Thus, within broad limits, when portal vein blood flow decreases, hepatic arterial blood flow increases. This hepatic arterial buffer response to decreasing portal blood flow maintains total blood flow to the liver at near-normal levels. This autoregulatory response of the hepatic artery is mediated by local release of adenosine, which vasodilates arterioles, lowers vascular resistance, and enhances arterial blood flow.

Hepatic blood volume is also quite large, amounting to one eighth of the total blood volume in the body. With various stresses, half of the hepatic reservoir of blood (375 ml in a 70-kg human adult) can be mobilized rapidly and propelled into the central circulation. Normal, although uncommon, stresses include heavy exercise and fright; pathological stresses include such disorders as hemorrhage and septic shock. The hepatic reserve volume is marshaled as part of the venous return to the heart and lungs after constriction of hepatic venules by sympathetic neural release of norepinephrine. A comparison of hepatic blood volume with that of other splanchnic organs and other bodily systems that can be mobilized by stress appears in Figure 8–2.

Gastric Circulation

The circulation of the stomach is influenced by the major function of the organ—namely, secretion of acid gastric juice—as well as by other neurohumoral factors previously discussed. In the 2 hrs surrounding a meal, 2 million oxyntic cells in the adult gastric mucosa may secrete 400 ml of a 0.1N HCl solution. This feat requires complex active transport processes at the apical membrane and extensive intracellular metabolic events to generate and extrude protons and Cl^- against large concentration gradients. Not surprisingly, there is a positive correlation between the rate of gastric acid secretion and the rate of gastric mucosal oxygen consumption. The gastric mucosal circulation continually provides oxygen, glucose, and fatty acids to fuel the active transport mechanisms, generates ATP, and energizes the intracellular enzymes required for secretion of acid gastric juice (see Chapter 2). The circulation also delivers water needed for the considerable volume of gastric juice being secreted (up to 2 L/24 hr in an adult male).

At normal or subnormal blood flows to the stomach, there is a positive correlation between an increase in the acid secretory rate and an increase in gastric mucosal blood flow (or, conversely, a decrease in secretion and blood flow). At high mucosal blood flow rates, changing secretory activity may not be accompanied by corresponding blood flow changes, because there is ample blood flow to meet the metabolic needs of the secreting mucosa. When a secretagogue, such as gastrin, stimulates secretion of acid gastric juice, the accompanying increase in mucosal blood flow is elicited by local vasodilator substances, such as adenosine, prostaglandins E and I, histamine, and NO.

Both gastric secretion and blood flow are controlled by autonomic neural regulators. The four nerve types that influence gastric mucosal blood flow are supplied by the sympathetic, parasympathetic, enteric, and primary sensory systems. Sympathetic fibers reach the stomach in either perivascular nerve trunks or vagi, release norepinephrine, and constrict gastric arterioles, thereby reducing mucosal blood flow. Parasympathetic fibers are delivered in the vagi, synapse with enteric nerve plexuses, and evoke release of acetylcholine. Acetylcholine is a vasodilator agent that acts directly on mucosal arterioles and stimulates oxyntic cell secretion of HCl, which raises mucosal metabolism and thereby indirectly elicits an increase in blood flow. The enteric nerves in the myenteric and submucosal plexuses release vasodilator neurotransmitters, such as acetylcholine, enkephalins, and VIP. Primary afferent nerves release vasodilator peptides, such as CGRP and substance P. The gastric mucosal arterioles are normally relatively relaxed, but this tonic state is reversed after vagotomy, which provokes vasoconstriction and reduced blood flow.

Topically applied agents that damage the gastric mucosal epithelium (e.g., aspirin, ethanol) cause an increase in the permeability of the mucosa to backdiffusion of HCl from the lumen into the tissue. The acid backdiffusion is accompanied by an increase in mucosal blood flow mediated by local primary afferent nerves that release CGRP. This local hyperemic response is a defense mechanism that carries off the backdiffusing acid and the injurious agent.

The gastric mucosal circulation can also be altered by vigorous contractions of the stomach wall. Brisk gastric motor activity will transiently decrease mucosal blood flow. The endothelial lining of the mucosal microcirculation produces agents that change blood flow. Endothelium-derived vasoactive factors include dilator agents such as NO, prostacyclin, and bradykinin and constrictor agents such as endothelin-1 and endothelin-2.

PATHOPHYSIOLOGY OF INTESTINAL ISCHEMIA

Ischemia is an abnormally low blood flow to an organ that persists sufficiently long to provoke functional or morphological evidence of cellular injury. In certain vital areas of the body (e.g., in cerebral or coronary arteries), even short bouts of ischemia can be life-threatening. Although the bowel is not as sensitive to acute reductions in blood flow as the heart or the brain, protracted superior mesenteric artery ischemia is incompatible with life. Intestinal ischemia may accompany other generalized circulatory disorders such as oligemic shock, ischemia in multiple organs, or congestive cardiac failure. Low-flow states of the gut may also occur as the result of intrinsic mesenteric circulatory disease (e.g., thrombotic occlusion of a superior mesenteric arterial branch). In addition, the syndrome of nonocclusive intestinal ischemia involves vasospasm in the superior mesenteric artery or one of its major branches and is often fatal.

A unique structural feature of the small intestinal microcirculation makes its mucosa especially vulnerable to the ravages of protracted ischemia. In this mucosal microcirculation, there is usually a central arteriole that runs the length of the villus. At the villus tip, the arteriole gives rise to a cascade of capillaries that course just beneath the basement membranes of the enterocytes. This arrangement allows rapid oxygenation of the absorptive cells that line the surface of the villus. The confluence of capillaries forms the venule still within the villus core near its base. Here the arteriole and venule are in close proximity (20 μm apart), with blood flowing in opposite directions in these vessels. Conditions are suitable for the diffusion of a lipid-soluble substance from the arteriole to the venule if the substance is in higher concentration in the arteriole than in the venule.

Oxygen physically dissolved in the plasma is one such substance, so that the gas diffuses from the arteriole into the venule, thereby short-circuiting the capillaries. This oxygen countercurrent exchange causes a concentration gradient for oxygen from the base of the villus to the tip, where the pO_2 is the lowest. Normally, this gradient is about 3 mm Hg and is of minor consequence, because villus blood flow is ample, and most of the oxygen is bound to hemoglobin in erythrocytes. However, in low-flow states, intestinal ischemia is compounded by the foregoing oxygen countercurrent exchange, and this exchange is exaggerated by the slowed velocity of blood perfusing the villus microcirculation. The result is that the oxygen gradient is also exaggerated, and death comes first to the enterocytes at the villus tip, where cells have the highest metabolic rate, are most vulnerable to hypoxic insult, and are the first to undergo necrosis in protracted nonocclusive intestinal ischemia (Fig. 8–16).

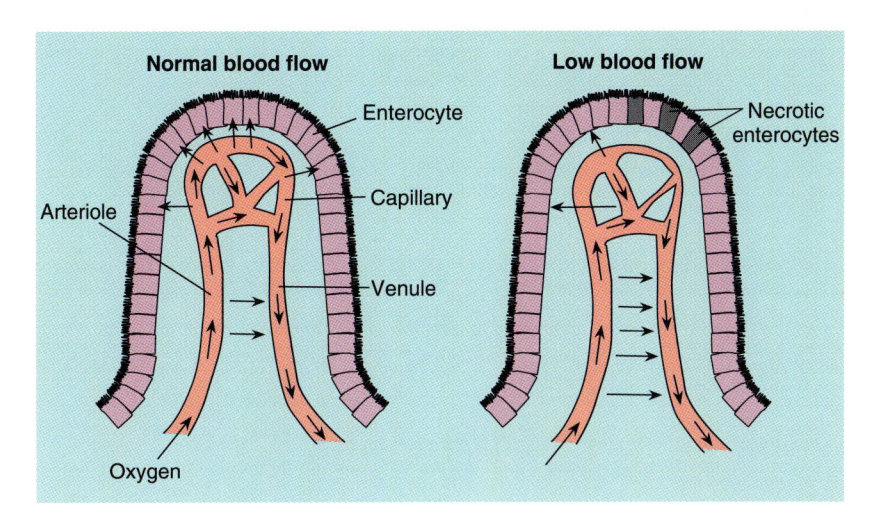

FIGURE 8–16. The oxygen countercurrent exchanger exaggerates the hypoxic insult to the villus tip during ischemic states. Lipid-soluble oxygen is shunted from the arteriolar plasma to the venular plasma in the lower villus shaft. With normal blood flow, there is an oxygen gradient from the base (higher pO_2) to the tip of the villus. In low-flow states, this gradient is exaggerated and intensifies hypoxia at the tip, causing necrosis of enterocytes.

The events that ensue in nonocclusive intestinal ischemia are portrayed in Figure 8–17. The patient is typically elderly, suffering from congestive cardiac failure, and receiving multiple drugs, including cardiac glycosides. Digitalis provokes mesenteric vasoconstriction through its peripheral adrenergic receptor stimulation. Heart failure contributes to the intestinal low-flow state because of the reduced cardiac output and elevated circulating angiotensin II levels that are the hallmarks of this disease. As intestinal ischemia worsens, the oxygen countercurrent mechanism comes into play, and the hypoxic insult to enterocytes causes cell death. With slowed mucosal blood flow velocity, microthrombi form and further increase resistance to blood flow. The dying intestinal epithelium loses one of its major functions: containment of luminal contents within the lumen. A variety of highly toxic organic materials penetrate the dysfunctional epithelial barrier and enter the dying circulation. Some absorbed noxious materials include bacterial endotoxins and enterotoxins, lysosomal hydrolases and cathepsins, and cytoplasmic components from disrupted enterocytes. The superimposition of massive toxemia on an elderly patient with heart failure and severe intestinal ischemia leads to irreversible shock. Without early diagnosis and adequate treatment, this syndrome is usually fatal.

In addition to nonocclusive intestinal ischemia, there are other disorders that reduce splanchnic blood flow (Fig. 8–18). In addition to occlusive diseases of the mesenteric arteries (e.g., thrombi, emboli), splanchnic blood flow also declines with certain other intrinsic digestive tract disorders (e.g., cirrhosis of the liver). In cirrhosis, the fibrotic liver obstructs portal blood flow and elevates portal pressure. Profound extrinsic circulatory states such as congestive cardiac failure and oligemic shock also compromise splanchnic blood flow.

Many steps involved in cell death from ischemia have been clarified (Fig. 8–19). Ischemic hypoxia provokes some anaerobic reactions in the intestinal mucosa that lead to cell death. Normal conversion of ATP to adenosine and resynthesis of ATP from adenosine is diminished, because adenosine is metabolized into hypoxanthine. Hypoxia also

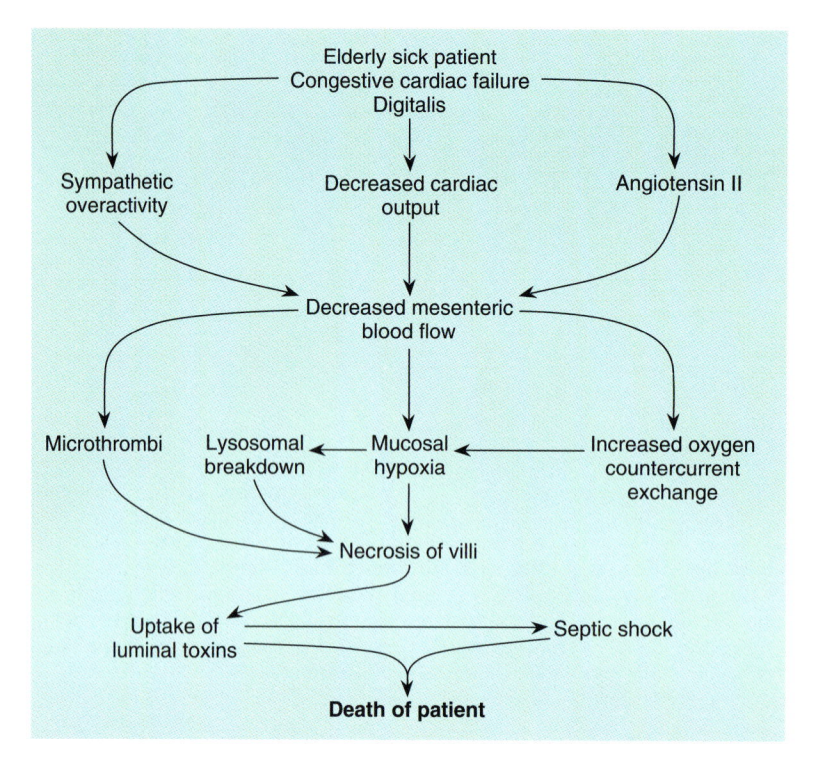

FIGURE 8–17. The pathogenesis of lethal nonocclusive intestinal ischemia. The major events are sequential and involve protracted ischemic hypoxia, epithelial necrosis, toxemia, irreversible shock, and death.

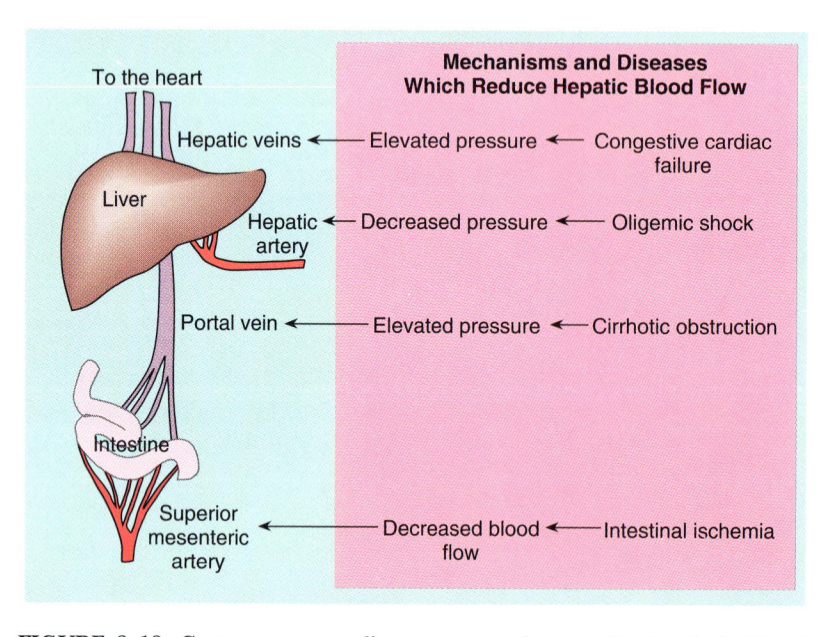

FIGURE 8–18. Common severe diseases cause decreased splanchnic blood flow. Congestive cardiac failure and hepatic cirrhosis increase venous pressure by obstructing blood flow out of the splanchnic circulation. Oligemic shock and intestinal ischemia decrease blood flow into the liver.

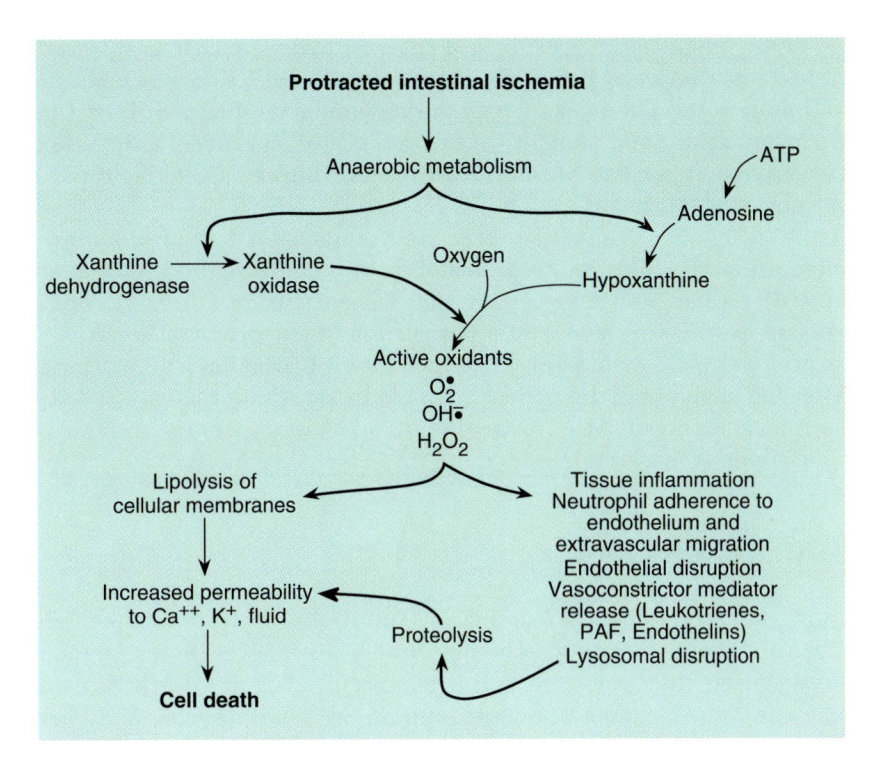

FIGURE 8–19. Ischemic hypoxia evokes active oxidant production, which leads to cell death. Anaerobic metabolism causes conversion of adenosine into hypoxanthine, which is the substrate for active oxidants. These cytotoxic agents induce acute inflammation, additional hypoxia, lipolysis, and proteolysis, leading to loss of cell membrane integrity and cell death. PAF indicates platelet activating factor.

converts xanthine dehydrogenase into xanthine oxidase. During the hypoxic insults, there are periods of reperfusion of the ischemic tissue with blood containing oxygen. Xanthine oxidase generates free radicals from hypoxanthine and oxygen in the mucosa. These active oxidants include oxygen free radical and hydrogen peroxide. These two oxidants combine to form the hydroxyl radical in a reaction facilitated by Fe^{+++} from hemoglobin; hydroxyl radical is especially cytotoxic. These active oxidants precipitate adhesion of neutrophils to the microvascular endothelium and the migration of neutrophils and erythrocytes from the vascular compartment into the extracellular space.

Cell membrane lipolysis occurs with production of leukotrienes and increased permeability of the membrane to ions and organic molecules. Lysosomes are disrupted, releasing proteolytic enzymes. Ca^{++} floods into cells, and key enzymatic reactions slow down. Vascular congestion and disrupted blood vessels are widespread, as is the death of a large proportion of the parenchymal cells. Advances in the development of free oxidant scavengers for therapeutic use provide the possibility of interrupting this pathological process before frank necrosis becomes widespread.

CASE REPORT: CONCLUSION

CLINICAL IMPRESSION. Mesenteric angina. Taken in isolation from the rest of the history, the patient's pain might have been considered dyspeptic except that the pain was located at the umbilicus, suggesting a small intestinal source. It was possible that the patient had a partial small bowel obstruction (e.g., Crohn's disease), but the absence of vomiting and the onset of pain during a meal implied a different etiology or a high obstruction. This pain, along with the presence of significant atherosclerotic disease, was strongly suggestive of intestinal ischemia, thus necessitating rapid evaluation to prevent infarction.

RECOMMENDATIONS. A small bowel series was obtained 1 hr after a meal and demonstrated thickened folds in the proximal small bowel distal to the ligament of Treitz. This led to a mesenteric angiogram that showed diffuse atherosclerotic disease in the aorta and iliac arteries and a 90% obstruction of the proximal superior mesenteric artery. A balloon angioplasty reduced this obstruction of the arterial lumen to 50%. After the angioplasty the patient was able to eat without pain, but 3 months later his symptoms recurred. After discussion, the patient underwent a successful bypass of the superior mesenteric artery.

CLINICAL OVERVIEW

According to careful postmortem analyses, up to 3% of deaths in general hospitals exhibit evidence of acute intestinal ischemia. Numerous reports attest to the difficulty of making this diagnosis (preoperatively and antemortem). The diagnostician is confronted with a subtle clinical presentation and several possible causes of acute abdomen.

Most commonly the patient suffering from an acute mesenteric ischemic crisis is elderly and has coexistent severe cardiovascular disease, especially congestive cardiac failure being treated with cardiac glycosides. Some unusual cardiovascular and nonvascular disorders that may contribute to the pathogenesis of mesenteric ischemia include subacute bacterial endocarditis, endocardial thrombi within the heart, use of predisposing agents (e.g., estrogen, cocaine, amphetamine), hypercoagulable states, myeloproliferative disease, vasculitides (e.g., polyarteritis nodosa, lupus erythematosus), and postvascular surgery for abdominal aneurism associated with inferior mesenteric arterial occlusion. Patients commonly present with an initial severe abdominal pain but without signs of an acute surgical abdomen (no rebound tenderness, audible bowel sounds, no intraperitoneal free air).

Successful diagnosis of life-threatening intestinal ischemia depends on a high degree of clinical suspicion. The abdominal radiograph may show "thumbprinting" of the bowel wall (intramural edema), intramural air, or portal venous air (usually a late sign). Diagnosis prior to exploratory surgery requires selective angiography. High-grade obstruction diagnosed with the use of a superior mesenteric arteriogram may offer the opportunity for interventional angioplasty, surgical bypass, or resection. In nonocclusive intestinal ischemia, some success has been achieved using intra-arterial infusion of mesenteric vasodilator drugs such as papaverine or prostaglandin E_1. Usually, however, such cases require surgical resection of the infarcted bowel.

REFERENCES

Several texts have appeared that should satisfy the special needs of some readers for more detailed information. These texts fall into two categories: medical physiology texts that either contain several chapters on gastrointestinal physiology or deal exclusively with this subject; and extensive treatises with dozens of chapters that review a broad range of topics in the biology of the digestive system.

Medical Physiology of the Gastrointestinal Tract

1. Fondacaro JD. Gastrointestinal physiology. In: Sperelakis N, Banks RO, eds. Physiology. Little, Brown, Boston, 1993.
2. Johnson LR. Gastrointestinal physiology. In: Johnson LR, ed. Essential Medical Physiology. Raven Press, New York, 1992.
3. Johnson LR, ed. Gastrointestinal Physiology. 4th ed. Mosby-Year Book, St. Louis, 1991.

Extensive Reviews of Gastrointestinal Tract Physiology

1. Johnson LR, ed. Physiology of the Gastrointestinal Tract. 3rd ed. Raven Press, New York, in press.
2. Schultz SG, ed. Handbook of Physiology. 2nd ed. American Physiological Society, Bethesda, MD, 1989.

INDEX

Note: Page numbers in *italics* refer to illustrations.

Absorption, 59. See also *Digestion*.
   amino acid, 81
   barriers to, 59–60, *60*
   calcium, *97*, 97–98
      dysfunctional, 98
      negative feedback mechanisms in, *97*, 97–98
   carbohydrate, 74, 76, 78–79
   cobalamin (vitamin B$_{12}$), *100*, 100–101
   disorders of. See *Malabsorption*.
   electrolyte, 61, *61*. See also *Sodium*.
   enzymes inhibiting, *68*, 68–69
   fat (lipid), 86, *88*
      defective, 88–89, *90*
   fluid, 61, *61*, 63, *63*, 67
      reduced, diarrhea associated with, 67–68
   fructose, 79
   galactose, 79
   glucose, 76, *78*, 78–79
   inhibition of, *68*, 68–69
   insufficient intestinal mucosal surface for, 89, *90*
   interprandial, *61*
   iron, 95–96, *96*
      effects of gastrectomy on, 103
      iron loss vs., 94–95
      negative feedback mechanisms in, 95–96, *96*
   lipid (fat), 86, *88*
      defective, 88–89, *90*
   mineral, physiology of, 94
   postprandial, 61, *61*, 64
   protein, 74, 79, 81
   salt (solute), transport and, 61, *61*. See also *Sodium*.
   sodium, 63, 67, 69. See also *Sodium, transport of*.
      glucose and, 70, 79
      postprandial, *61*, 64
      reduced, diarrhea associated with, 67–68
   sodium chloride, inhibition of, *68*, 68–69
   solute, transport and, 61, *61*. See also *Sodium*.
   tryptophan, defective, 81
   vitamin, physiology of, 94
   vitamin A, 101–102, *102*
   vitamin B$_{12}$ (cobalamin), *100*, 100–101
   water, 61, *61*, 63, *63*, 67
      reduced, diarrhea associated with, 67–68
Acetylcholine, effects of, on gastric secretion, 31–32, 36, *36*
   on pancreatic secretion, 49, *50*, 52, *53*, 54
   on smooth muscle cell contraction, 3, *5*
   on splanchnic circulation, 112
Achalasia, 21, *22*
Acid secretion, by stomach, 29–38
   adenylate cyclase and, 31, *32*
   blood flow and, 119
   calcium and, 31, *32*, *33*, 34
   cephalic phase of, 36, *36*
      suppression of, 37, *38*
   control of, 34–38

Acid secretion (Continued)
   cyclic AMP and, 31, *33*, 34
   enzyme effects and, 31, *32*, *33*, 34, *35*
   esophagitis due to, 9
   gastric phase of, *36*, 36–37
   inhibition of or protection against, 31, *32*, *37*, 37–38, 55
   intestinal phase of, *36*, 37
   secretagogue effects on oxyntic cells and, 31–36, *33*, *34*, *36*
Acinar cells, pancreatic, 46
   alpha-amylase production in, 49
   carboxypeptidase production in, 51
      protein breakdown in relation to, 51, 80, *80*
   electrolyte and water secretion by, *51*, 52
   enzymes produced in, 49–51, 56
      insufficiency of, 45, 55, 56
      lipid digestion by, 50, 85, *85*, 86, 87
      protein degradation by, 51, 80, *80*
      secretory mechanisms and, 48–49, *49*, *50*
      starch degradation by, 49
   lipase production in, 50
      fat digestion in relation to, 50, 85, *85*, 86, 87
      insufficiency of, 55
   trypsin production in, 50–51
      protein breakdown in relation to, 51, 80, *80*
Actin, 3
Adenosine, effects of, on intestinal blood flow, 117, *118*
Adenosine monophosphate, cyclic, and gastric acid secretion, 31, *33*, 34
Adenylate cyclase, and gastric acid secretion, 31, *32*
Alcohol abuse, pancreatic disease due to, 91
Alpha-amylase, 49
   degradation of starch by, 49, 75, *75*, 76
Alpha cells, glucagon secretion by, 46
Alpha-limit dextrins, 74
Amino acids, absorption of, 81
   breakdown of proteins into, 80, *80*
   transport of, 81, *81*
      defects in, 81
Aminoaciduria, 81
AMP, cyclic, and gastric acid secretion, 31, *33*, 34
Anal sphincter, external, 18, *19*
Anemia, clinical overview of, 103
   iron deficiency and, 95, 103
   malabsorption and, 82
   pernicious, 40, 99, 103
   possible causes of, 103
      in patient with Crohn's ileitis, 103
   vitamin B$_{12}$ deficiency and, 99
Angina, mesenteric, 105, 123–124. See also *Mesenteric circulation*.
   causes of, 120–121, *121* *123*, 123
Antiabsorptive enzymes, *68*, 68–69
Arterioles, effects of norepinephrine on, *109*
   myogenic properties of, 115

127

Arterioles (Continued)
   resistance at, 108, *108*
Atrophy, of intestinal villi, 82
Autonomic nerves, vasoactive neurotransmitters released by, *111*
   response of splanchnic circulation to, 110–113, *114*
Autoregulatory mechanisms, in splanchnic circulation, 112, *113*, 114

Bacterial overgrowth, in ileum, 104
   Crohn's disease and, 103
Beta cells, insulin secretion by, 47
   deficiency of or insensitivity to, 46
Beta-carotene, in gastrointestinal processing of vitamin A, 101, 102
Bicarbonate (HCO$_3$) secretion, by pancreas, 51–52, *52*, *53*
Bile salts, lipid emulsification by, 84
   micelle formation with lipids by. See *Micelle(s)*.
Biopsy, of small intestine, in diagnosis of cause of malabsorption, 82
Bleeding, gastrointestinal, anemia due to, 103
   response of splanchnic circulation to, 110, *111*
Blood flow. See *Circulation*.
Blue diaper syndrome, 81
Bowel. See *Colon; Small intestine*.

CA-19-9 levels, in pancreatic cancer, 91
Calcium, 96
   absorption of, *97*, 97–98
      dysfunctional, 98
      negative feedback mechanisms in, *97*, 97–98
   accumulation of, and gastric acid secretion, 31, 32, *33*, 34
   in response to norepinephrine, *109*, 112, *112*
   concentration of, and smooth muscle cell contraction, 3, *5*, *6*
   deficiency of, 98
   excess of, 98
   plasma levels of, response of parathyroid gland to, 97
   recommended daily allowance for, 96
   saponification of, 98
   solubilization of, 96
      failure of, 98
   sources of, 96
cAMP (cyclic adenosine monophosphate), and gastric acid secretion, 31, *33*, 34
Cancer, pancreatic, 46, 90–91
   case report of, 83, 89–90
   clinical overview of, 90–91
   fat maldigestion in, 90
   levels of CA-19-9 in, 91
   metastasis of, 91
   steatorrhea in, 90
Capacitance vessels, venules as, *108*
Capillaries, exchange at, *108*
Carbohydrate(s), 74
   absorption of, 74, 76, 78–79
   digestible, 74
   digestion of, 74, *75*, 76
      effects of lactase deficiency on, 76–77, *77*
   energy provided by, 74

Carbohydrate (s) (Continued)
   indigestible, 74
   metabolism of, physiology of, 74
   sources of, 74
Carbonic anhydrase, and gastric acid secretion, 34, *35*
Carboxypeptidase, 51
   breakdown of proteins by, 51, 80, *80*
Celiac artery, blood flow in, *106*
   changes in, possible causes of, 106–107
Celiac sprue, 82
Cephalic phase, of gastric secretion, 36, *36*
   suppression of, 37, *38*
   of pancreatic secretion, 54
Chewing, 6
Children, lactase deficiency in, effects of, 76–77
Chloride, concentration of, in pancreatic juice, 52, *53*
   secretion of, by crypt cells, and diarrhea, 68, 69, 70
   transport of, in and out of oxyntic cells, *30*, 31
Cholecystokinin, 53–54
   effects of, on pancreatic secretion, 49, *50*, 52, 53, *53*, 54
   gastrin vs., 54
Cholera, 69
   diarrhea in, 69, 70, *70*
   treatment of, 70, *70*
Cholesterolester hydrolase, lipid digestion by, *87*
Chronic pancreatitis, pain in, 91
Chylomicrons, 88
   in gastrointestinal processing of vitamin A, 102
Chyme, 14
   mixing of, *15*, 17
   propulsion of, *15*
      into duodenum, 11, *12*, 13
Circulation, 105–124
   gastric, 119–120
   hepatic, 118–119
      blood flow in, *106*
   intestinal. See *Circulation, mesenteric*.
   mesenteric, 115–117
      arterioles in, *108*
         effects of norepinephrine on, *109*
      blood flow in, *106*
         intestinal oxygen consumption vs., 117, *118*
         postprandial increase in, 116
      capillaries in, *108*
      conditions compromising, 120–121, *121–23*, 123
         case report of, 105, 123–124
         clinical overview of, 124
      effects of norepinephrine on, *109*, 112, *113*
      endothelial nitric oxide release in, 115, *116*
      microscopic vessels in, *108*
      venules in, *108*
   pancreatic, 46, *47*
   splanchnic, 105–115
      autoregulatory mechanisms in, 112, *113*, 114
      blood flow in, *106*, 106–107
         control of, 109–115, *110*, *117*
         decreased vascular resistance to, 109, *110*
         increased vascular resistance to, 109, *109*
         total body blood volume in relation to, 107, *107*
         vascular resistance to, 108, *108*
      conditions compromising, 121, *122*
      hemodynamics of, 108–109

Circulation (Continued)
  myogenic properties of arterioles and, 115
  physiology of, 105–115
  response of, to autonomic nerves and their vasoactive neurotransmitters, 110–113, *111, 114*
    to enhanced postprandial metabolism, 113–114, *115*
    to hemorrhage, 110, *111*
    to nitric oxide, 115, *116*
    to nonadrenergic, noncholinergic vasodilator nerves, 112–113, *114*
    to norepinephrine, *109,* 112, *112, 113*
Cobalamin (vitamin B$_{12}$), 98–99
  absorption of, *100,* 100–101
  binding of, to intrinsic factor, 39, 99, *100*
    to nonintrinsic factor cobalophilins, 99
  deficiency of, 99, 100, 103–104
    clinical overview of, 103–104
  gastrointestinal processing of, 99–101, *100*
  hepatic sites of, 99
  metabolic functions of, 99
  recommended daily allowance for, 99
  sources of, 99
Colipase, facilitating effect of, on digestion of fat by lipase, 85, *85*
Colon, 17–18
  blood supply to. See *Circulation, mesenteric.*
  mass movement in, 19, *19*
  peristalsis in, 18
  rhythmic segmentation in, 19
  sodium absorption in, 67
    reduced, diarrhea associated with, 67–68
  sodium transport in, 66–67, *67*
  unabsorbed tryptophan in, fate of, 81
  undigested lactose in, effects of, 77, *77*
  undigested wheat starch in, fate of, 77
  water absorption in, 67
    reduced, diarrhea associated with, 67–68
Concentration gradient, in transcellular transport, 61, *62*
Constipation, 20
  case report of, 2, 21
  clinical overview of, 21, 23
Contractility, smooth muscle, 3, *5, 6*
Crohn's disease, case report of, 93–94, 103
  causes of anemia in, 103
  ileal stricture in, 103
  overgrowth of ileal bacteria in, 103
Crypt cells, intestinal, 58, *59,* 66
  chloride secretion by, and diarrhea, 68, 69, 70
Cyclic AMP, and gastric acid secretion, 31, *33,* 34
Cyclic nucleotides, in vascular smooth muscle cells, effects of, *109, 110*
Cystic fibrosis, and pancreatic insufficiency, 55
Cytoprotective effects, of prostaglandins, 41

Defecation, 20
  reduced frequency of, 20
    case report of, 2, 21
    clinical overview of, 21, 23
Delta cells, gastrin secretion by, 47
    excessive, 47–48
Diabetes mellitus, 46
Diarrhea, 68–70

Diarrhea (Continued)
  case report of, 57, 70–71
  chloride secretion by crypt cells and, 68, 69, 70
  cholera and, 69, 70, *70*
  clinical overview of, 71
  Escherichia coli enterotoxin and, 69
  infectious, 69, 71
    case report of, 57, 70–71
    clinical overview of, 71
  inhibition of absorption and, *68,* 68–69
  lactase deficiency and, 77, *77*
  osmotic, 68
  reduced sodium or water absorption and, 67–68
  secretory, 68
    case report of, 57, 70–71
    cholera and, 69, 70, *70*
    clinical overview of, 71
    crypt cells in, 68, 69, 70
    Escherichia coli enterotoxin and, 69
    inhibited sodium chloride absorption and, *68,* 68–69
  traveler's (turista), 69
    case report of, 57, 70–71
  treatment of, 70, 71
Diffusion, 61, *62*
  paracellular, 60–61, *61*
  passive, of sodium, into enterocytes, 63, *64*
Digestible carbohydrates, 74
Digestion. See also *Absorption.*
  carbohydrate, 74, *75,* 76
    effects of lactase deficiency on, 76–77, *77*
  disorders of. See *Maldigestion.*
  effects of enzyme deficiency on, 55, *56*
  fat. See *Digestion, lipid.*
  lactose, 76
    defective, 76–77, *77*
      case report suggestive of, 73
  lipid, 84
    cholesterolester hydrolase in, *87*
    defective, 88, *89*
      pancreatic disease and, 55, 90
    emulsification in, 84
    lipase in, 50, 85, *85, 86, 87*
      colipase and, 85, *85*
    micelles in, 84, 86, *86, 88*
    pancreatic enzymes in, 50, 85, *85, 86, 87*
    phospholipase A$_2$ in, *87*
  milk, 76
    defective, 76–77, *77*
      case report suggestive of, 73
  protein, 51, 74, 79, 80, *80*
  starch, 49, *75,* 75–76, *76*
  sucrose, 76
  wheat starch, incomplete, 77
Dipeptidases, breakdown of proteins by, *80*
Disaccharidases, breakdown of starch digestion products by, 76. See also *Carbohydrate(s)* and *Starches.*
Duct cells, pancreatic, 46
  bicarbonate (HCO$_3^-$) secretion by, 51–52, *52, 53*
Duodenum. See also *Stomach.*
  propulsion of chyme into, 11, *12,* 13
  rhythmic segmentation in, 13
  ulcer of, 41, 42, 43
    case report of, 25, 42
    clinical overview of, 42–43
    pain due to, 25, 42

Duodenum (Continued)
   vitamin B$_{12}$ binding to intrinsic factor in, 100

Eating, absorption following, 61, *61,* 64
   chewing in, 6
   enhanced metabolism following, response of splanchnic circulation to, 113–114, *115*
   gastric secretion in response to, 36–37, *36–38*
   increased intestinal blood flow following, 116
   pancreatic secretion in response to, 52, *52,* 54
   swallowing in, 6
      control of, 8–9, *10*
      esophageal response to, 8, *9*
      oropharyngeal phase of, *7,* 7–8
Electrical gradient, in transcellular transport, 61, *62*
Electrolyte(s). See also specific substances, e.g., *Sodium.*
   absorption of, 61, *61*
   diffusion of, paracellular, 60–61, *61*
   secretion of, gastric, 34, *35*
      pancreatic, *51,* 52
   transport of, transcellular, *61,* 61–62, *62*
Electrolyte solutions, glucose-containing, in treatment of diarrhea, 70, *71*
Emulsification, of fats, 84
Endocrine pancreas, gastrin secretion by, 47
      excessive, 47–48
   glucagon secretion by, 46
   hormone secretion by, 46–48
   insulin secretion by, 47
      deficiency of or insensitivity to, 46
   polypeptide secretion by, 48
   somatostatin secretion by, 48
Endopeptidases, breakdown of proteins by, 80, *80*
Endothelial release, of nitric oxide, in mesenteric circulation, 115, *116*
Energy, carbohydrates as source of, 74
   fats as source of, 84
Enteric nervous system, 2, 8–9, 16, 18
Enterocyte(s), 58, *59*
   calcium absorption in, *97,* 97–98
      dysfunctional, 98
      negative feedback mechanisms and, *97,* 97–98
   cobalamin (vitamin B$_{12}$) absorption in, *100,* 100–101
   effects of ischemia on, 120, *121*
   fat (lipid) absorption in, 86, *88*
   fat (lipid) resynthesis in, 87–88, *89*
   fatty acid–binding proteins in, 87
   fructose absorption in, 79
   galactose absorption in, 79
   glucose absorption in, 76, 78–79
   inhibition of absorption in, *68,* 68–69
   interprandial absorption in, *61*
   iron absorption in, 95–96, *96*
      effects of gastrectomy on, 103
      iron loss vs., 94–95
      negative feedback mechanisms and, 95–96, *96*
   lipid (fat) absorption in, 86, *88*
   lipid (fat) resynthesis in, 87–88, *89*
   microvilli of, 58, *59*
      carbohydrate digestion at, 76
      protein digestion at, 80, *80*
      surface area provided by, 58
         loss of, 98
   mineral absorption in, 94

Enterocyte(s) (Continued)
   Na$^+$,K$^+$-ATPase (sodium pump) in, 62, 64, 65, 66, 79
   paracellular diffusion around, 60–61, *61*
   postprandial absorption in, 61, *61*
   site of, 58, *59.* See also *Small intestine.*
   sodium pump (Na$^+$,K$^+$-ATPase) in, 62, 64, 65, 66, 79
   sodium transport by, 64, *64,* 65, *65,* 66
   transcellular transport across, 61, *61,* 62
   vitamin absorption in, 94
   vitamin A processing in, 101–102, *102*
   vitamin B$_{12}$ (cobalamin) absorption in, *100,* 100–101
Enterotoxins, as cause of diarrhea, 69
Enzymes, antiabsorptive, *68,* 68–69
   contributory effects of, in gastric acid secretion, 31, 32, *33,* 34, *35*
   effects of deficiency of, on digestion, 55, *56*
   lipid digestion by, 50, 85, *85, 86, 87*
   pancreatic. See *Pancreas, enzymes produced in.*
   protein degradation by, 51, 80, *80*
      and breakdown of protein digestion products, 81
   starch degradation by, 49, 75, *75, 76*
      and breakdown of starch digestion products, 76. See also *Carbohydrate(s)* and *Starches.*
Escherichia coli enterotoxin, as cause of diarrhea, 69
Esophagitis, peptic, 9
Esophagus, 8
   achalasia of, 21, *22*
   lower sphincter of, 8, 9, *9*
   motor disorders of, 21, *22*
   pain in, 1, 21
   muscle cells of, control of, 8, *11*
   peristaltic wave in, 8, 9
   reflux of gastric acid into, 9
   response of, to swallowing, 8, *9*
      control of, 8, *10*
   spasm of, 21, *22*
      case report of, 1–2, 20
      clinical overview of, 21
   upper sphincter of, 8, *9*
Exchange vessels, capillaries as, *108*
Exocrine pancreas, alpha-amylase production in, 49
   bicarbonate (HCO$_3^-$) secretion by, 51–52, *52, 53*
   carboxypeptidase production in, 51
      protein breakdown in relation to, 51, 80, *80*
   electrolyte and water secretion by, *51,* 52
   enzymes produced in, 49–51, *56*
      insufficiency of, 45, 55, *56*
      lipid digestion by, 50, 85, *85, 86, 87*
      protein degradation by, 51, 80, *80*
      secretory mechanisms and, 48–49, *49, 50*
      starch degradation by, 49
   function of, control of, 49, *50, 53,* 53–55
   lipase production in, 50
      fat digestion in relation to, 50, 85, *85, 86, 87*
      insufficiency of, 55
   secretagogues affecting, 49, *50,* 52, 53, *53,* 54
   trypsin production in, 50–51
      protein breakdown in relation to, 51, 80, *80*
Exopeptidases, breakdown of proteins by, 80, *80*
External anal sphincter, 18, *19*

Fat(s), 84

Fat (s) (Continued)
  absorption of, 86, *88*
    defective, 88–89, *90*
  bile salt micelle formation with. See *Micelle(s)*.
  digestion of, 84
    cholesterolester hydrolase in, *87*
    defective, 88, 89
      pancreatic disease and, 55, 90
    emulsification in, 84
    lipase in, 50, 85, *85, 86, 87*
      colipase and, 85, *85*
    micelles in, 84, 86, *86, 88*
    pancreatic enzymes in, 50, 85, *85, 86, 87*
    phospholipase A² in, *87*
  emulsification of, 84
  energy provided by, 84
  fecal, 89
    malabsorption and, 82, 89
    pancreatic cancer and, 90
    pancreatic insufficiency and, 55, 56
  malabsorption of, 88–89, *90*
  maldigestion of, 88, 89
    pancreatic disease and, 55, 90
  metabolism of, physiology of, 84–88
  resynthesis of, 87–88, *89*
  satiety value of, 84
  sources of, 85
Fat-soluble vitamins, 98. See also *Vitamin A*.
Fatty acid–binding proteins, in enterocytes, 87
Feces, excretion of, 20
    reduced frequency of, 20
      case report of, 2, 21
      clinical overview of, 21, 23
  fat in, 89
    malabsorption and, 82, 89
    pancreatic cancer and, 90
    pancreatic insufficiency and, 55, 56
  protein in, 79–80
  water in, excessive. See *Diarrhea*.
Ferric iron, reduction of, to ferrous iron, 95
Ferritin, 95
Ferrous iron, binding of, to storage protein, 95
    to transport protein, 95
  reduction of ferric iron to, 95
  release of, from heme, 95
Fibrosis, cystic, pancreatic insufficiency in, 55
Fluid(s), absorption of, 61, *61*, 63, *63*, 67
    reduced, diarrhea associated with, 67–68
  diffusion of, paracellular, 60–61, *61*
  excretion of, *63*
    excessive, in stools. See *Diarrhea*.
  ingestion of, *63*
  osmosis of, 61
  secretion of, gastrointestinal, *63*
    pancreatic, *51*, 52
  transport of, transcellular, 61, *61*Food consumption. See *Eating*.
Fructose, absorption of, 79
  intolerance of, case history suggestive of, 73

G protein(s), 3
  inhibitory, 31
  stimulatory, 31
Galactose, absorption of, 79
Gastrectomy, effects of, on iron absorption, 103
Gastric acid secretion, 29–38

Gastric acid secretion (Continued)
  adenylate cyclase and, 31, *32*
  blood flow and, 119
  calcium and, 31, 32, *33*, 34
  cephalic phase of, 36, *36*
    suppression of, 37, *38*
  control of, 34–38
  cyclic AMP and, 31, *33*, 34
  enzyme effects and, 31, 32, *33*, 34, *35*
  esophagitis due to, 9
  gastric phase of, *36*, 36–37
  inhibition of or protection against, 31, *32*, 37, 37–38, 55
  intestinal phase of, *36*, 37
  secretagogue effects on oxyntic cells and, 31–36, *33, 34, 36*
Gastric circulation, 119–120
Gastric emptying, 12–15, *14*
Gastric juice, *28*, 29, 34. See also *Stomach*.
  hydrochloric acid in. See *Gastric acid secretion*.
  intrinsic factor in, 39–40, 99
    binding of cobalamin (vitamin B₁₂) to, 39, 99, 100
    reduced secretion of, effects of, 103–104
  ionic concentrations in, 34, *35*
  mucus in, 29, 39
  pepsin in, 39, *40*
    breakdown of proteins by, 80, *80*
Gastric pacemaker, 11
  slow waves and spike potentials elicited by, 11, 12, *13*
Gastric peristalsis, 10, 11, 12, *12, 13*, 14
  slow waves and, 11, 12, *13*
  spike potentials and, 11, *13*
Gastric phase, of acid secretion by stomach, *36*, 36–37
  of juice secretion by pancreas, 54
Gastric retropulsion, 11, *12*
Gastrin, 47
  cholecystokinin vs., 54
  effects of, on gastric acid secretion, 31–32, 36, *36*, 37
  excessive secretion of, 47–48
Gastrin-releasing peptide, 36, 37
Gastritis, 41
Gastroesophageal reflux, 9
Gastrointestinal tract, bleeding from, anemia due to, 103
  fluid secretion by, *63*
  motility of, 2–23. See also *Peristalsis*.
    disorders of, 21, *22*, 23, *23*
      case reports of, 1–2, 20–21
      clinical overview of, 21, 23
    physiology of, 2–20
    smooth muscle contractility and, 3, *5, 6*
  postprandial function of. See *Eating*.
  protein degradation in, 80, *80*
  smooth muscle cells of, 3, *4*
    contractility of, 3, *5, 6*
    organization of, *4*, 5
    relaxation of, 4
  starch degradation in, 75, *75*
  vitamin A processing in, 101–102, *102*. See also *Vitamin A*.
  vitamin B₁₂ (cobalamin) processing in, 99–101, *100*. See also *Vitamin B₁₂ (cobalamin)*.
Glucagon, 47

Glucose, absorption of, 76, *78*, 78–79
Glucose-containing electrolyte solutions, in treatment of diarrhea, 70, 71
Gluten exclusion diet, for celiac sprue, 82
Goblet cells, intestinal, 58, *59*

H_2 receptor antagonists, 31
Hartnup's disease, 81
HCl secretion, by stomach. See *Hydrochloric acid secretion, by stomach.*
HCO_3^- (bicarbonate) secretion, by pancreas, 51–52, *52, 53*
Heme, release of ferrous iron from, 95
Hemochromatosis, 95, 96
Hemorrhage, gastrointestinal, anemia due to, 103
  response of splanchnic circulation to, 110, *111*
Hepatic circulation, 118–119
  blood flow in, *106*
Hepatocytes, vitamin A in, 102
  vitamin B_{12} (cobalamin) in, 99
Hirschsprung's disease, anorectal manometric findings in, *23*
Histamine, effects of, on gastric acid secretion, 31, 35, 36, *36*, 37
H^+,K^+-ATPase (proton pump), and gastric acid secretion, 31, 32, *33*, 34, *35*
Hormone secretion, by pancreas, 46–48
  by parathyroid gland, 97
Hydrochloric acid secretion, by stomach, 29–38
  adenylate cyclase and, 31, *32*
  blood flow and, 119
  calcium and, 31, 32, *33*, 34
  cephalic phase of, 36, *36*
    suppression of, 37, *38*
  control of, 34–38
  cyclic AMP and, 31, *33*, 34
  enzyme effects and, 31, 32, *33*, 34, *35*
  esophagitis due to, 9
  gastric phase of, *36*, 36–37
  inhibition of or protection against, 31, *32*, *37*, 37–38, 55
  intestinal phase of, *36*, 37
  secretagogue effects on oxyntic cells and, 31–36, *33, 34, 36*
Hypercalcemia, 98
Hyperemia, postnorepinephrine, *113*
  postprandial, 116
Hypervitaminosis A, 102, 103
Hypocalcemia, 98
Hypoxia, ischemic, 121, 123, *123*

IF. See *Intrinsic factor.*
Ileitis, Crohn's, case report of, 93–94, 103
Ileocecal sphincter, *18*
Ileum. See also *Small intestine.*
  bacterial overgrowth in, 104
    Crohn's disease and, 103
  Crohn's disease of, case report of, 93–94, 103
  enterocytes of, inhibition of absorption in, *68*, 68–69
  transport of sodium by, *65*
  resection of, effects of, 89, 104
  stricture of, Crohn's disease and, 103
  vitamin B_{12} (cobalamin) absorption in, *100*, 100–101
Indican, conversion of tryptophan to, 81

Indigestible carbohydrates, 74
Infants, lactase deficiency in, effects of, 76–77
  newborn, Hartnup's disease (blue diaper syndrome) in, 81
Infectious diarrhea, 69, 71
  case report of, 57, 70–71
  clinical overview of, 71
Inhibitory G protein, 31
Inorganic (bicarbonate [HCO_3^-]) secretion, by pancreas, 51–52, *52, 53*
Inorganic (hydrochloric acid [HCl]) secretion, by stomach. See *Hydrochloric acid secretion, by stomach.*
Insulin, 47
  deficiency of or insensitivity to, 46
Interprandial absorption, *61*
Interprandial secretion, of gastric juice, *28,* 29, 34
  of pancreatic juice, *51,* 52, 54
Intestinal circulation. See *Mesenteric circulation.*
Intestinal phase, of gastric secretion, *36,* 37
  of pancreatic secretion, 54
Intestine. See *Colon; Small intestine.*
Intolerance, fructose, case history suggestive of, 73
  lactose, 76–77
    case history suggestive of, 73
Intrinsic factor, 39–40, 99
  binding of vitamin B_{12} (cobalamin) to, 39, 99, 100
  reduced secretion of, effects of, 103–104
Iron, 94
  absorption of, 95–96, *96*
    effects of gastrectomy on, 103
    iron loss vs., 94–95
    negative feedback mechanisms in, 95–96, *96*
  deficiency of, 95, 103
  excess of, 95, 96
  ferric, reduction of, to ferrous iron, 95
  ferrous, binding of, to storage protein, 95
    to transport protein, 95
    reduction of ferric iron to, 95
    release of, from heme, 95
  loss of, 94–95
  recommended daily allowance for, 95
  sources of, 95
Ischemia, 120
  hypoxia due to, 121, 123, *123*
  intestinal, 120–121, *121–123*, 123. See also *Mesenteric circulation.*
    case report of, 105, 123–124
    clinical overview of, 124
Islet cells, 46
  gastrin secretion by, 47
    excessive, 47–48
  glucagon secretion by, 46
  hormone secretion by, 46–48
  insulin secretion by, 47
    deficiency of or insensitivity to, 46
  polypeptide secretion by, 48
  somatostatin secretion by, 48

Kwashiorkor, 79

Lactase, deficiency of, effects of, 76–77, *77*
  case report suggestive of, 73
Lactose, digestion of, 76
  defective, 76–77, *77*

Lactose (Continued)
  case report suggestive of, 73
Large intestine. See *Colon.*
Lipase, 50
  fat digestion by, 50, 85, *85, 86, 87*
  insufficient secretion of, effects of, 55
Lipid(s). See *Fat(s).*
Liver, circulation in, *106,* 118–119
  vitamin A in, 102
  vitamin B$_{12}$ (cobalamin) in, 99
Lower esophageal sphincter, 8, 9, *9*

Malabsorption, 82
  case report of, 73–74, 82
  clinical overview of, 82
  fat, 88–89, *90*
  steatorrhea as sign of, 82, 89
Maldigestion, diagnosis of, 82
  fat, 88, 89
    pancreatic disease and, 55, 90
  lactose, 76–77, *77*
    case report suggestive of, 73
Maltose, 74
Maltotriose, 74
Mesenteric circulation, 115–117
  arterioles in, *108*
    effects of norepinephrine on, *109*
  blood flow in, *106*
    intestinal oxygen consumption vs., 117, *118*
    postprandial increase in, 116
  capillaries in, *108*
  conditions compromising, 120–121, *121–123,* 123
    case report of, 105, 123–124
    clinical overview of, 124
  effects of norepinephrine on, *109,* 112, *113*
  endothelial nitric oxide release in, 115, *116*
  microscopic vessels in, *108*
  venules in, *108*
Micelle(s), formation of, 84
  in digestion of lipids, 84, 86, *86,* 88
  in gastrointestinal processing of vitamin A, 101
Microvilli, of enterocytes, 58, *59.* See also *Enterocyte(s).*
  carbohydrate digestion at, 76
  protein digestion at, 80, *80*
  surface area provided by, *58*
    loss of, 98
Migrating motor complex, 15, 16
Milk, digestion of, 76
  defective, 76–77, *77*
    case report suggestive of, 73
Minerals. See also *Calcium* and *Iron.*
  absorption of, physiology of, 94
Motility, gastrointestinal, 2–23. See also *Peristalsis.*
  disorders of, 21, *22,* 23, *23*
    case reports of, 1–2, 20–21
    clinical overview of, 21, 23
  physiology of, 2–20
  smooth muscle contractility and, 3, *5, 6*
Mouth, movement of food from, to stomach, 6–9, *7, 9, 10*
Mucous cells, gastric, 27, *27,* 29
Mucus, gastric, 29, 39
Muscle, esophageal, control of, 8, *11*

Muscles (Continued)
  small intestinal, 16
  smooth, cells of, 3, *4*
    contraction of, 3, *5, 6*
    effects of cyclic nucleotides in, 109, *110*
    influence of nitric oxide on, 115, *116*
    organization of, *4, 5*
    relaxation of, 4
Myogenic properties, of arterioles, 115
Myosin, 3

Na$^+$,K$^+$-ATPase (sodium pump), 29, 51, 62, 64, 65, 66, 79. See also *Sodium.*
Nausea, 15
Nervous system, autonomic, vasoactive neurotransmitters released by, *111*
    response of splanchnic circulation to, 110–113, *114*
  enteric, 2, 8–9, 16, 18
Newborn, Hartnup's disease (blue diaper syndrome) in, 81
Nitric oxide (NO), influence of, on vascular smooth muscle cells, 115, *116*
Nonadrenergic, noncholinergic vasodilator nerves, 112
  response of splanchnic circulation to, 112–113, *114*
Nonintrinsic factor cobalophilins, 99
Norepinephrine, autoregulatory response to, 112, *113*
  vasoconstrictor effects of, *109,* 112, *112*
Nucleotides, cyclic, in vascular smooth muscle cells, effects of, 109, *110*

Oral rehydration solutions, in treatment of diarrhea, 71
Organic (enzyme) secretion, by pancreas, 48–51, *49, 50*
  and lipid digestion, 50, 85, *85, 86, 87*
  and protein degradation, 51, 80, *80*
  and starch degradation, 49
  insufficiency of, 45, 55, 56
Organic (IF, mucus, pepsin) secretion, by stomach, 39–40. See also *Oxyntic cells, intrinsic factor secretion by; Pepsin.*
Oropharynx, movement of food through, 6, 7, *7,* 8
  control of, 8–9, *10*
  esophageal response to, 8, *9*
Osmosis, 61
Osmotic diarrhea, 68
Oxygen consumption, vs. blood flow, in intestine, 117, *118*
Oxyntic cells, 27, *27, 28,* 29
  chloride transport in and out of, *30,* 31
  hydrochloric acid secretion by. See *Hydrochloric acid secretion.*
  intrinsic factor secretion by, 39–40, 99
    binding of vitamin B$_{12}$ (cobalamin) in relation to, 39, 99, *100*
    effects of reduction in, 103–104
  potassium transport into, 29, *30*
  secretagogues affecting, 31–36, *33, 34, 36*
  sodium transport out of, 29, *30*

Pacemaker, gastric, 11
    slow waves and spike potentials elicited by, 11, 12, *13*
Pain, in chronic pancreatitis, 91
  in esophageal motor disorders, 1, 21
  in intestinal ischemia, 105, 123–124
  in peptic ulcer disease, 25, 42
Pancreas, 45, 46
  acinar cells of, 46
    alpha-amylase production in, 49
    carboxypeptidase production in, 51
      protein breakdown in relation to, 51, 80, *80*
    electrolyte and water secretion by, *51,* 52
    enzymes produced in, 49–51, 56
      insufficiency of, 45, 55, 56
      lipid digestion by, 50, 85, *85, 86, 87*
      protein degradation by, 51, 80, *80*
      secretory mechanisms and, 48–49, *49, 50*
      starch degradation by, 49
    lipase production in, 50
      fat digestion in relation to, 50, 85, *85, 86, 87*
      insufficiency of, 55
    trypsin production in, 50–51
      protein breakdown in relation to, 51, 80, *80*
  alpha-amylase production in, 49
  alpha cells of, glucagon secretion by, 46
  anatomy of, 46, *47*
  beta cells of, insulin secretion by, 47
    deficiency of or insensitivity to, 46
  bicarbonate (HCO$_3^-$) secretion by, 51–52, *52, 53*
  blood supply to, 46, *47*
  cancer of, 46, 90–91
    case report of, 83, 89–90
    clinical overview of, 90–91
    fat maldigestion in, 90
    levels of CA-19-9 in, 91
    metastasis of, 91
    steatorrhea in, 90
  carboxypeptidase production in, 51
    protein breakdown in relation to, 51, 80, *80*
  cell types in, 46
  delta cells of, gastrin secretion by, 47
    excessive, 47–48
  disease of, 46, 90–91
    case reports of, 45, 55, 83, 89–90
    clinical overview of, 55–56, 90–91
    fat maldigestion in, 55, 90
    history of alcohol abuse and, 91
    steatorrhea in, 55, 56, 90
  duct cells of, 46
    bicarbonate (HCO$_3^-$) secretion by, 51–52, *52, 53*
  electrolyte and water secretion by, *51,* 52
  endocrine, gastrin secretion by, 47
    excessive, 47–48
    glucagon secretion by, 46
    hormone secretion by, 46–48
    insulin secretion by, 47
      deficiency of or insensitivity to, 46
    polypeptide secretion by, 48
    somatostatin secretion by, 48
  enzymes produced in, 49–51, 56
    insufficiency of, 45, 55, 56
    lipid digestion by, 50, 85, *85, 86, 87*
    protein degradation by, 51, 80, *80*
    secretory mechanisms and, 48–49, *49, 50*
    starch degradation by, 49
  exocrine, alpha-amylase production in, 49

Pancreas (Continued)
  bicarbonate (HCO$_3^-$) secretion by, 51–52, *52, 53*
  carboxypeptidase production in, 51
    protein breakdown in relation to, 51, 80, *80*
  electrolyte and water secretion by, *51,* 52
  enzymes produced in, 49–51, 56
    insufficiency of, 45, 55, 56
    lipid digestion by, 50, 85, *85, 86, 87*
    protein degradation by, 51, 80, *80*
    secretory mechanisms and, 48–49, *49, 50*
    starch degradation by, 49
  function of, control of, 49, *50, 53,* 53–55
  lipase production in, 50
    fat digestion in relation to, 50, 85, *85, 86, 87*
    insufficiency of, 55
  secretagogues affecting, 49, *50,* 52, 53, *53,* 54
  trypsin production in, 50–51
    protein breakdown in relation to, 51, 80, *80*
  function of, control of, 49, *50, 53,* 53–55
  gastrin secretion by, 47
    excessive, 47–48
  glucagon secretion by, 46
  HCO$_3^-$ (bicarbonate) secretion by, 51–52, *52, 53*
  hormone secretion by, 46–48
  inflammation of, 46
    chronic, pain in, 91
  innervation of, 46, *47*
  inorganic (bicarbonate [HCO$_3^-$]) secretion by, 51–52, *52, 53*
  insufficient enzyme secretion by, 55, 56
    case history of, 45, 55
    clinical overview of, 55–56
    cystic fibrosis and, 55
  insulin secretion by, 47
    deficiency of or insensitivity to, 46
  islet cells of, 46
    gastrin secretion by, 47
      excessive, 47–48
    glucagon secretion by, 46
    hormone secretion by, 46–48
    insulin secretion by, 47
      deficiency of or insensitivity to, 46
    polypeptide secretion by, 48
    somatostatin secretion by, 48
  lipase production in, 50
    fat digestion in relation to, 50, 85, *85, 86, 87*
    insufficiency of, 55
  organic (enzyme) secretion by, 48–51, *49, 50*
    and lipid digestion, 50, 85, *85, 86, 87*
    and protein degradation, 51, 80, *80*
    and starch degradation, 49
    insufficiency of, 45, 55, 56
  peptide hormones secreted by, 46–48
  physiology of, 45–56
  polypeptide secretion by, 48
  secretagogues affecting, 49, *50,* 52, 53, *53,* 54
  somatostatin secretion by, 48
  trypsin production in, 50–51
    protein breakdown in relation to, 51, 80, *80*
  tumors of, hormone-secreting, 47, 48
    malignant. See *Pancreas, cancer of.*
  water and electrolyte secretion by, *51,* 52
Pancreatic insufficiency, 55, 56
  case history of, 45, 55
  clinical overview of, 55–56
  cystic fibrosis and, 55
Pancreatic juice, 45

Pancreatic juice (Continued)
    bicarbonate (HCO$_3^-$) in, 51–52, *52, 53*
    chloride in, 52, *53*
    electrolytes and water in, *51*, 52
    enzymes in, 49–51, 56
        insufficiency of, 45, 55, 56
        lipid digestion by, 50, 85, *85, 86, 87*
        protein degradation by, 51, 80, *80*
        secretion of, 48–49, *49, 50*
        starch degradation by, 49
    secretion of, 53–55
        cephalic phase of, 54
        control of, 49, *50, 53*, 53–55
        gastric phase of, 54
        interprandial, *51*, 52, 54
        intestinal phase of, 54
        postprandial, 52, *52*, 54
        protective effects of, 55
Pancreatic polypeptide, 48
Pancreatitis, 46
    chronic, pain in, 91
Paracellular diffusion, 60–61, *61*
Parathyroid gland, response of, to plasma levels of calcium, 97
Parietal cells. See *Oxyntic cells.*
Pepsin, breakdown of proteins by, 80, *80*
    secretion of, 39, *40*
Peptic cells, 27, *27*, 29
Peptic esophagitis, 9
Peptic ulcer, 41, 42, 43
    case report of, 25, 42
    clinical overview of, 42–43
    pain due to, 25, 42
Peptide hormones, pancreatic secretion of, 46–48
Peristalsis, 6–7
    in colon, 18
    in esophagus, 8, 9
    in pharynx, 8
    in rectum, 18
    in small intestine, 15–17
    in stomach, 10, 11, 12, *12, 13*, 14
        slow waves and, 11, 12, *13*
        spike potentials and, 11, *13*
        rhythmic segmentation vs., *15*
Pernicious anemia, 40, 99, 103
Pharynx, peristaltic wave in, 8
Phospholipase A$_2$, lipid digestion by, *87*
Pinocytosis, 62
Polypeptide, pancreatic, 48
Portal vein, blood flow in, *106*, 118
Postnorepinephrine hyperemia, *113*
Postprandial gastrointestinal function. See *Eating.*
Potassium, transport of, into oxyntic cell, 29, *30*
Prostaglandins, cytoprotective effects of, 41
Protein(s), 79
    absorption of, 74, 79, 81
    deficiency of, 79
    digestion of, 51, 74, 79, 80, *80*
    fatty acid–binding, in enterocytes, 87
    fecal, 79–80
    G, 3
        inhibitory, 31
        stimulatory, 31
    metabolism of, physiology of, 74
    storage, binding of ferrous iron to, 95
    transport, binding of ferrous iron to, 95

Protein kinases, and gastric acid secretion, 31, 32, *33*
    and inhibition of absorption, 68, 69
Proton pump (H$^+$,K$^+$-ATPase), and gastric acid secretion, 31, 32, *33*, 34, *35*
Pylorus, obstruction of, 43

Receptive relaxation, of stomach, 8
Recommended daily allowance, for calcium, 96
    for iron, 95
    for vitamin A, 101
    for vitamin B$_{12}$ (cobalamin), 99
Rectum, 20
    function of, 20
        manometric studies of, *23*
    peristalsis in, 18
Reflux, gastroesophageal, 9
Rehydration solutions, oral, in treatment of diarrhea, 71
Resistance vessels, arterioles as, 108, *108*
Resynthesis, lipid, 87–88, *89*
Retinaldehyde, in gastrointestinal processing of vitamin A, 101, *102*
Retinoids, 101. See also *Vitamin A.*
Retinyl esters, in gastrointestinal processing of vitamin A, 101, *102*
Retropulsion, in stomach, 11, *12*
Rhythmic segmentation, colonic, 19
    duodenal, 13
    mixing of chyme in, *15, 17*
    peristalsis vs., *15*

Salt (solute) transport, 60–62, *61, 62.* See also *Sodium.*
Saponification, of calcium, 98
Satiety value, of fats, 84
Schilling test, 104
Second-messenger systems, and gastric acid secretion, 31, *33*
    and inhibition of absorption, *68*, 68–69
Secretagogue(s), 31
    acetylcholine as, 31–32, 36, *36*, 49, *50, 52, 53*, 54
    cholerystokinin as, 49, *50, 52, 53, 53*, 54
    gastrin as, 31–32, 36, *36*, 37
    histamine as, 31, 35, 36, *36*, 37
    secretin as, 49, *50, 52, 53, 53*, 54
Secretin, effects of, antacid, 55
    pancreatic secretory, 49, *50, 52, 53, 53*, 54
Secretory diarrhea, 68
    case report of, 57, 70–71
    cholera and, 69, 70, *70*
    clinical overview of, 71
    crypt cells in, 68, 69, 70
    Escherichia coli enterotoxin and, 69
    inhibited sodium chloride absorption and, *68*, 68–69
Segmentation, rhythmic, colonic, 19
    duodenal, 13
    mixing of chyme in, *15, 17*
    peristalsis vs., *15*
Slow waves, and gastric peristalsis, 11, 12, *13*
Small intestine, 57–60
    amino acid absorption in, 81
    bacterial overgrowth in, 104
        Crohn's disease and, 103

Small intestine (Continued)
　barriers to absorption in, 59–60, *60*
　biopsy of, in diagnosis of cause of malabsorption, 82
　calcium absorption in, *97,* 97–98
　　dysfunctional, 98
　　negative feedback mechanisms and, *97,* 97–98
　carbohydrate absorption in, 74, 76, 78–79
　carbohydrate digestion in, 74, 75, 76
　　effects of lactase deficiency on, 76–77, *77*
　cell turnover in, 58
　cell types in, 58, *59.* See also *Enterocyte(s).*
　cobalamin (vitamin B$_{12}$) absorption in, *100,* 100–101
　Crohn's disease of distal portion of, case report of, 93–94, 103
　crypt cells of, 58, *59,* 66
　　chloride secretion by, and diarrhea, 68, 69, 70
　electrolyte absorption in, 61, *61.* See also *Small intestine, sodium absorption in.*
　electrolyte transport in, 60–62, *61.* See also *Small intestine, sodium transport in.*
　enterocytes of. See *Enterocyte(s).*
　fat absorption in, 86, *88*
　　defective, 88–89, *90*
　fat digestion in, 84
　　cholesterolester hydrolase and, *87*
　　colipase and, 85, *85*
　　defective, 88, 89
　　　pancreatic disease and, 55, 90
　　emulsification and, 84
　　lipase and, 85, *85, 86, 87*
　　micelles and, 84, 86, *86, 88*
　　pancreatic enzymes and, 85, *85, 86, 87*
　　phospholipase A$_2$ and, *87*
　fat resynthesis in, 87–88, *89*
　fluid absorption in, 61, *61,* 63, *63*
　folds of Kerckring in, *58*
　fructose absorption in, 79
　galactose absorption in, 79
　glucose absorption in, 76, *78,* 78–79
　goblet cells of, 58, *59*
　inadequate mucosal absorptive surface in, 89, *90*
　instillation of glucose-electrolyte solutions into, as treatment for diarrhea, 70, 71
　interprandial absorption in, *61*
　iron absorption in, 95–96, *96*
　　effects of gastrectomy on, 103
　　iron loss vs., 94–95
　　negative feedback mechanisms and, 95–96, *96*
　ischemia of, 120–121, *121–123,* 123. See also *Mesenteric circulation.*
　　case report of, 105, 123–124
　　clinical overview of, 124
　lactose digestion in, 76
　　defective, 76–77, *77*
　　　case report suggestive of, 73
　lipid digestion and absorption in. See S*mall intestine, fat absorption in; Small intestine, fat digestion in.*
　lipid resynthesis in, 87–88, *89*
　milk digestion in, 76
　　defective, 76–77, *77*
　　　case report suggestive of, 73
　mineral absorption in, 94
　motility of, 15–17
　muscle in, 16

Small intestine (Continued)
　paracellular diffusion in, 60–61, *61*
　peristalsis in, 15–17
　physiology of, 57–60
　postprandial absorption in, 61, *61,* 64
　protein absorption in, 74, 79, 81
　protein digestion in, 74, 79, 80, *80*
　protein loss from, 79–80
　resection of, effects of, 89, 104
　salt (solute) absorption in, 61, *61.* See also *Small intestine, sodium absorption in.*
　salt (solute) transport in, 60–62, *61.* See also *Small intestine, sodium transport in.*
　sodium absorption in, 63
　　glucose and, 79
　　postprandial, *61,* 64
　sodium transport in, 63–66, *64, 65*
　　apical membrane mechanisms and, 63–66, *64, 65*
　　basolateral membrane mechanisms and, 64, *64, 65,* 65, 66
　　crypt cell mechanisms and, 66
　　electrogenic mechanisms and, 64
　　electroneutral mechanisms and, 65, *65*
　　facilitation of amino acid absorption by, 81
　　facilitation of glucose absorption by, *78,* 78–79
　solute absorption in, 61, *61.* See also *Small intestine, sodium absorption in.*
　solute transport in, 60–62, *61.* See also *Small intestine, sodium transport in.*
　starch digestion in, *75,* 75–76
　stricture of, Crohn's disease and, 103
　sucrose digestion in, 76
　surface area of, 57, *58*
　transcellular transport in, 61, *61,* 62
　villi of, 57, 58, *58, 59.* See also *Enterocyte(s).*
　　atrophy of, 82
　　effects of ischemia on, 120, *121*
　vitamin absorption in, 94
　vitamin A processing in, 101–102, *102*
　vitamin B$_{12}$ (cobalamin) absorption in, *100,* 100–101
　water absorption in, 61, *61,* 63, *63*
　wheat starch digestion in, incomplete, 77
Smooth muscle cells, 3, *4*
　contraction of, 3, *5, 6*
　organization of, *4,* 5
　relaxation of, 4
　vascular, effects of cyclic nucleotide accumulation in, 109, *110*
　　influence of nitric oxide on, 115, *116*
Sodium, absorption of, 63, 67, 69
　glucose and, 70, 79
　postprandial, *61,* 64
　reduced, diarrhea associated with, 67–68
　transport of, colonic, 66–67, *67*
　　out of oxyntic cell, 29, *30*
　　small intestinal, 63–66, *64, 65*
　　　apical membrane mechanisms in, 63–66, *64, 65*
　　　basolateral membrane mechanisms in, 64, *64, 65,* 65, 66
　　　crypt cell mechanisms in, 66
　　　electrogenic mechanisms in, 64
　　　electroneutral mechanisms in, 65, *65*
　　　facilitation of amino acid absorption by, 81
　　　facilitation of glucose absorption by, *78,*

Sodium (Continued)
78–79
Sodium chloride, absorption of, inhibition of, *68*, 68–69
pancreatic acinar cell secretion of, *51*, 52
Sodium pump (Na+,K+-ATPase), 29, 51, 62, 64, 65, 66, 79
Solubilization, of calcium, 96
failure of, 98
Solutes. See also *Sodium*.
absorption of, 61, *61*
diffusion of, paracellular, 60–61, *61*
transport of, transcellular, *61*, 61–62, *62*
Somatostatin, 48
effects of, on gastric acid secretion, 38
Spasm, esophageal, 21, *22*
case report of, 1–2, 20
clinical overview of, 21
Sphincter(s), anal, external, 18, 19
esophageal, 8, 9, *9*
ileocecal, *18*
Spike potentials, and gastric peristalsis, 11, *13*
Splanchnic circulation, 105–115. See also *Circulation*.
autoregulatory mechanisms in, 112, *113*, 114
blood flow in, *106*, 106–107
control of total body blood volume in relation to, 107, *107*, 109-115, *110*, 117
vascular resistance to, 108
arterioles and, 108, *108*
decreased, 109, *110*
increased, 109, *109*
conditions compromising, 121, *122*
hemodynamics of, 108–109
myogenic properties of arterioles and, 115
physiology of, 105–115
response of, to autonomic nerves and their vasoactive neurotransmitters, 110–113, *111*, 114
to enhanced postprandial metabolism, 113–114, *115*
to hemorrhage, 110, *111*
to nitric oxide, 115, *116*
to nonadrenergic, noncholinergic vasodilator nerves, 112–113, *114*
to norepinephrine, *109*, 112, *112*, *113*
Sprue, celiac, 82
Starches, 75. See also *Carbohydrate(s)*.
dietary, 74
digestion of, 49, *75*, 75–76, *76*
wheat, incomplete digestion of, 77
Steatorrhea, 89
malabsorption and, 82, 89
pancreatic cancer and, 90
pancreatic insufficiency and, 55, 56
Stimulatory G protein, 31
Stomach, 9, 26–27
acid secretion by, 29–38
adenylate cyclase and, 31, *32*
blood flow and, 119
calcium and, 31, 32, *33*, 34
cephalic phase of, 36, *36*
suppression of, 37, *38*
control of, 34–38
cyclic AMP and, 31, *33*, 34
enzyme effects and, 31, 32, *33*, 34, *35*
esophagitis due to, 9
gastric phase of, *36*, 36–37
inhibition of or protection against, 31, *32*, 37,

Stomach (Continued)
37–38, 55
intestinal phase of, *36*, 37
secretagogue effects on oxyntic cells and, 31–36, *33*, *34*, *36*
anatomy of, *26*, 26–27
cell types in, 26, 27, *27*
circulation in, 119–120
diseases of, 25, 40–43
distention of, acid secretion in response to, 36–37
emptying of, 12–15, *14*
hydrochloric acid secretion by. See *Stomach, acid secretion by*.
inflammatory (peptic) diseases of, 25, 40–43
inorganic (hydrochloric acid [HCl]) secretion by. See *Stomach, acid secretion by*.
intrinsic factor secretion by, 39–40, 99
binding of vitamin B$_{12}$ (cobalamin) in relation to, 39, 99, 100
effects of reduction in, 103–104
movement of food to, from mouth, 6–9, *7*, *9*, *10*
mucosal injury to, 40–42, *41*
mucous cells of, 27, *27*, 29
mucus secreted by, 29, 39
obstruction of pyloric outflow of, 43
organic (IF, mucus, pepsin) secretion by, 39–40. See also *Stomach, intrinsic factor secretion by*; *Stomach, pepsin secretion by*.
oxyntic cells of, 27, *27*, *28*, 29
chloride transport in and out of, *30*, 31
hydrochloric acid secretion by. See *Stomach, acid secretion by*.
intrinsic factor secretion by. See *Stomach, intrinsic factor secretion by*.
potassium transport into, 29, *30*
secretagogues affecting, 31–36, *33*, *34*, *36*
sodium transport out of, 29, *30*
pacemaker of, 11
slow waves and spike potentials elicited by, 11, 12, *13*
parietal cells of. See *Stomach, oxyntic cells of*.
pepsin secretion by, 39, *40*
breakdown of proteins in relation to, 80, *80*
peptic cells of, 27, *27*, 29
peptic diseases of, 25, 40–43
peristalsis in, 10, 11, 12, *12*, *13*, 14
slow waves and, 11, 12, *13*
spike potentials and, 11, *13*
physiology of, 26–42
receptive relaxation of, 8
reflux of contents of, into esophagus, 9
resection of, effects of, on iron absorption, 103
retropulsion in, 11, *12*
secretagogues affecting, 31–36, *33*, *34*, *36*
Stool, excretion of, 20
reduced frequency of, 20
case report of, 2, 21
clinical overview of, 21, 23
fat in, 89
malabsorption and, 82, 89
pancreatic cancer and, 90
pancreatic insufficiency and, 55, 56
protein in, 79–80
water in, excessive. See *Diarrhea*.
Storage protein, binding of ferrous iron to, 95
Stricture, ileal, Crohn's disease and, 103
Sucrose, digestion of, 76

Swallowing, 6
    control of, 8–9, *10*
    esophageal response to, 8, *9*
    oropharyngeal phase of, *7*, 7–8
Swallowing center, 8, *10*

Transcellular transport, *61*, 61–62, *62*

response of splanchnic circulation to, 112–113, *114*
Venules, as capacitance vessels, *108*
Vibrio cholerae infection, 69
    diarrhea in, 69, 70, *70*
    treatment of, 70, *70*
Villi, intestinal, 57, 58, *58, 59*. See also *Enterocyte(s)*.
    atrophy of, 82

Zollinger-Ellison syndrome, 47–48